THE FARM

Other books by Grace Olson

The Yard
Merlin Finds His Magic

graceolsonauthor.com

THE FARM

MY JOURNEY DEEPENS

GRACE OLSON

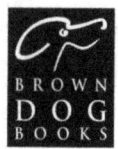

BROWN
DOG
BOOKS

Published under licence by Brown Dog Books and The Self-Publishing Partnership Ltd, 10b Greenway Farm, Bath Rd, Wick, nr. Bath BS30 5RL, UK

www.selfpublishingpartnership.co.uk

ISBN printed book: 978-1-83952-782-1
ISBN e-book: 978-1-83952-783-8

Cover design by Andrew Prescott
Cover image: 'Two Hearts' watercolour on Langton board © Ruth Buchanan 2023
Internal design by Andrew Easton

Printed and bound in the UK

This book is printed on FSC® certified paper

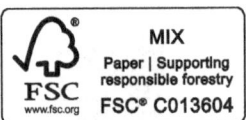

Dedication

I dedicate this book to all horses everywhere.
Thank you for tolerating humans with such
grace and dignity.

Chapter 1

I woke up in a cold sweat. My heart was racing and felt like it was almost bursting out of my chest.

Oh my God! my mind shrieked. *What have I done?*

My alarm went off, which made me jump, even though I was already awake.

'Mummy! Wrexford has done a wee in the kitchen!' shouted my daughter, Florence, from down the stairs.

'Oh bloody hell,' I sighed, dragging my dressing gown on. I dashed to the kitchen to survey the damage. The morning whirlwind had begun. Urine trickled down the cupboard doors and formed a stinking yellow pool on the floor.

'Bloody dog,' I grumbled as I mopped it up with a load of kitchen towel.

Wrexford Whippet leaped around, wagging his tail completely oblivious of the extremely irritating situation that he had created. His smelly paws splatting extra wee all over the tiles. Thank God it wasn't carpet.

Eventually, after the chaos of cleaning up and making breakfast, Florence was deposited at school, Wrexford had been walked and the morning madness melted away. I breathed a deep sigh of relief.

Oh God. The horse. A sensation of nausea began to rise.

I wasn't working until the afternoon so I had time to go to the livery yard. Funny how this usually pleasant drive had suddenly reverted back to one of total anxiety, the way it had been when it all began last spring.

The yard was always quiet midweek early morning so I was alone as I hurried up the path to the horse field. I was armed with maracas in case the two feral ponies, who really shouldn't have been at a livery yard and created stress on a daily basis, decided to cause trouble – they were the last things I wanted to deal with today. Luckily, they were too busy snoozing to be interested in me so I was able to get to the gate without any harassment.

Poppy was quietly grazing far away from all the other horses. I stood and looked at her and felt a wave of sickness wash over me.

'Oh hell,' I said out loud.

'What's up, luv?' asked a familiar Yorkshire voice. I almost jumped out of my skin. I had been so caught up in my thoughts I hadn't noticed my friend Jack walking up the path behind me.

'Oh nothing much. Just feeling a bit weird.'

'You are a bit weird,' laughed Jack. 'Come on, get her headcollar on and let's get out of here before anyone else arrives. I've had an exciting idea.'

Jack leaped over the gate and hurried towards Buddy, her lovely, laid-back, skewbald cob. He was so chilled out she put his headcollar on and they ambled back over to the gate.

'Hello, Poppy,' I said as she looked at me with deep suspicion. 'Let's go for a nice walk.' I reached out to put her headcollar on and her ears went straight back.

'Ow! Why did you nip me? What's that about?' I rubbed my hand as she glowered at me. 'Come on now, let me put this on.' I reached up tentatively and once again she bared her teeth, but she let me fasten the headcollar without actually biting. I could feel my blood pressure begin to rise. 'Good girl, walk on.' Poppy didn't budge. 'Come on, Poppy,' I pleaded. Still nothing. 'Poppy!'

I shouted. Her eyes opened wide and a look of fear flitted across her face.

'Oh heck I'm sorry Poppy. Let's remember what I learned in Wales. What would Julie say? Just breathe and relax.' I paused and consciously let go of the tension in my arms. 'And breathe again to let it all out. Right, shall we go and have a nice trip out?' Poppy snorted and lowered her head. 'Great. Let's walk on.'

'Sorted?' laughed Jack as Poppy finally agreed to walk with me to the gate.

'She's hard work,' I sighed.

'I thought things had improved since the Wales thing?' asked Jack. 'Why was she biting you?'

'I don't know. She's been behaving really stressy again.'

'How strange,' mused Jack. 'Well let's crack on. Oh bugger, is that Amanda?'

'Who's Amanda?' I looked down the path to the yard where Jack was squinting at a forty-odd-year-old woman in a very smart business suit.

'Yes it is. Damn. That's all we need.'

Jack hurried down to the yard and Poppy and I trotted after her to meet the mysterious Amanda. It was unusual to see Jack so rattled.

'Hello, Jack,' greeted Amanda curtly. 'Who do we have here?' She peered over the top of her glasses and looked me up and down exactly like the headmistress from my primary school days.

'This is Grace. She bought Poppy from Bernie recently. Grace, this is Bob's daughter, Amanda.'

'Who's Bob?' I asked, having a bit of a brain fart.

'The yard owner,' Amanda replied sternly.

'Oh heck yes of course, sorry.' I bit my lip trying not to explode with nervous laughter.

'I'm here to remind everyone that winter rules will be enforced from next month,' said Amanda in a very no-nonsense manner. 'All the horses have to be out by eight a.m. and in by five p.m. A fine of one pound will be added to your bill each time you are late. That will be all. Enjoy your ride.' And with that she marched off towards the outdoor arena.

'For God's sake,' sighed Jack. 'She's such a miserable cow. Let's get tacked up.'

We groomed and tacked up at top speed and clattered out of the yard like the Charge of the Light Brigade.

'I can't get here for eight every morning,' I panicked when we were out of earshot.

'I can't get here for five p.m. either,' grumbled Jack. 'She's such a bitch. We have to get out of here. It was awful last winter.'

'And I can't afford to be fined. I can't even really afford to own a horse! Oh God, why have I done this?'

'Calm down, I've had an idea.' Jack looked like she meant business.

'Ok,' I replied while thinking, *Oh crikey what the hell has she come up with now?* Jack was prone to having wild ideas.

'What do you think about getting our own place?' asked Jack as we approached the cross road that would take us onto a bridle path.

'What do you mean?' I asked.

'Our own field. Wouldn't it be great to not have to deal with any of the mad rules in this place? It would really help with our expenses too.'

I ruminated on this as we rode down the bridle path into the village.

'How can this help with expenses? Won't it cost a fortune to buy our own land and build a stable block and everything else we'll need?'

'No.' Jack shook her head. 'We aren't buying the land. We just need to rent some, and we don't need stables either.'

'What do you mean we don't need stables? What will we do with the horses in winter?' I was aghast at such a suggestion and thought she had lost her mind.

'Horses don't need stables. Where in the wild would you ever see a horse standing in a shed?'

'Er ...'

'Exactly! You wouldn't see it because it's not natural. Horses don't want to be shut in. They want to be able to walk around even at night in winter.'

'I suppose you've got a point. But what if it's really bad weather? Won't they need somewhere to get away from that?'

'I will build us the best field shelter you've ever seen in your life,' declared Jack with tremendous passion. She loved building things and was a very skilful joiner. 'I've already designed it and I've been wanting to build one for years.'

I was discombobulated by the concept of the whole thing and didn't know what to say.

'We just need to find the right place,' she continued enthusiastically.

'We need to know how much it would cost first.' I had visions of it costing thousands.

'A mate of mine is renting ten acres in Shadwell and that's

only costing him a hundred pounds a month,' said Jack.

'A hundred pounds? That's so much less than what we're paying. Wow!'

'Yep! Wow!' Jack grinned.

'Well it's definitely worth looking into,' I conceded.

'Absolutely. Have a think about it and we can chat about it again, but we need to keep it quiet. Don't tell anyone because we don't want any shit from Bob's daughter if she knows we're thinking of leaving.'

'Ok.' I nodded.

We continued our ride through the quaint village without speaking for a while. I noticed none of its usual charm because my head was swimming with all the 'what ifs' of getting our own land coupled with all the 'what ifs' of suddenly being a horse owner.

'I think we should have a drive round to check out all the local empty fields,' said Jack, breaking the silence. 'Just to get an idea of what's out there.'

Finally, we wandered back into the yard and were greeted with quite a kerfuffle as the place was busying up with horse owners.

'Oh for goodness' sake, Brenda! I thought you were going to get those feral ponies of yours trained? They're a real menace. Look what they've done to my new rug!' Morag was holding up a horse rug with a giant tear down the middle.

'Oh bloody hell,' said Jack. 'How did that happen?'

'I'd only left it by the gate for literally two minutes and I came back to this!' Morag's eyes were popping out of her head in anger.

'I'm so sorry, Morag. I'll buy you another one,' squeaked Brenda, red-faced. Her unkempt mousy brown hair wafted around her face, which made her look even more fragile than usual.

'Well you'd better go and get one now because my horse is going to need a rug on tonight,' Morag snapped, witheringly. It was interesting to notice how her Scottish accent grew thicker the more irritated she became, and though only short and stocky, she appeared to be massive now that she was so furious. I could imagine how fearsome she must have been when she'd been in the army.

I leaped off Poppy and was just leading her into the barn to untack when I was stopped in my tracks.

'Grace!' Morag's foghorn voice boomed through my head at what felt like a hundred decibels. I could feel Poppy's heart jump from the sheer force of the volume. 'Poppy will need a rug it's going to be cold tonight!'

'Oh I er ...' I had no idea about horse rugs and hadn't thought to buy any.

'Oh blimey, it's going to be cold tonight. Which rug are you putting on Boudica?' called Noor to Danny, both of whom had just arrived.

'I'm not sure, it's not looking too bad. Maybe a fifty gram?' Danny pondered, looking at his phone.

'Fifty gram?' Noor studied her phone. 'My weather app says it's going to be six degrees with a twenty-two mile an hour westerly wind, no rain and real feel will be three degrees. Surely, they'll need at least a one hundred gram half neck?' she asked.

I had absolutely no idea what she was talking about.

'Really?' Morag chimed in, fumbling in her pocket for her phone. 'Well I've got the BBC app and it says it's going to be, let's see. Hang on a minute. Oh for goodness' sake it's taking its time to load. Ah here it is now, it's a seventy-five percent chance of heavy rain between two a.m. and six a.m. with a twenty-seven mile per hour northwesterly wind wind and real feel of one degree Centigrade. Hell's bells that calls for a two hundred and fifty gram rug with a full neck!'

I could feel my blood pressure begin to rise from the sheer embarrassment of my ignorance. What the heck were they talking about? What was a two hundred and fifty gram rug? And why would anyone have a weather app on their phone?

'Bloody glad I've got a cob,' muttered Jack as she walked past with Buddy, leading him back to the field with no rug. I watched Morag and Noor march off to their stables still discussing rugs.

'Does Poppy need a rug?' I wondered out loud as I led her over to her stable to untack her. I had never in my life had anything to do with horse rugs and I felt completely unfit to be a horse owner. My face was as red as a beetroot.

'Oh dear, Grace,' came the sickly-sweet voice of Louise. I hadn't noticed her watching us. As usual she was immaculately dressed as if ready for a show. 'You should have stuck to loaning other people's hairy cobs at that cheap yard you used to be at. If you don't know what a sports horse needs, do you really think you should own one?'

I felt like I'd been punched in the stomach and was too stunned to reply as Louise smirked, tossed her perfect golden curls over her shoulder and stalked off.

'Poppy will need quite a few rugs,' said Danny kindly, who had overheard Louise's cutting remarks. 'She'll need a fifty gram half neck rain sheet for when it's rainy but not too cold. A hundred gram maybe with a detachable neck for when it's a bit colder. Then probably a two-fifty gram combo for when it's heavy rain and below five degrees and windy and then when it's freezing and snowy I'd say a three-fifty or four hundred gram rug.'

My bottom jaw fell open as my brain went into meltdown. *Why on earth does she need so many rugs? And what the hell is a combo?*

'Ha! Don't panic! I'll take you rug shopping,' laughed the laid-back Danny when he saw my expression. He steered me and Poppy over to the chairs in the barn, sat me down and opened his phone.

'Right, here's a really cheap online horse shop. I'll order them for you and then just pay me back.' He grinned.

'What's a combo?' I hissed. I didn't mind Danny knowing of my ignorance but I didn't want anyone else to hear. He smiled and showed me a photo of an all-in-one horse rug with a neck cover.

'Some of them come with a neck that you can zip on and off,' he whispered, winking, as Morag strode over once again. She swiftly untacked Poppy and measured her with a tape measure that she produced from her pocket (why she had that in her pocket I have no idea). Danny sorted out every type of rug that Poppy would need. Rugs I had never heard of as the previous cobs I had loaned had been more than capable of growing their own winter coats.

'Poppy is so thin skinned she will need a rug,' explained Danny, pointing to Poppy's rump. 'Look at her thin tail and now look at how sparse her mane is. And look closely at her fur here on her back. It's very fine really, isn't it?'

'God yes, she's like my whippet,' I replied.

'Exactly,' agreed Danny. 'So this type of horse needs a rug. She's not as tough as a native breed like Buddy. She's a man-made breed. The sporty horses are usually rug wearers.'

Who knew? I had never considered the subject before but now I was a few hundred pounds lighter thanks to Poppy's rubbish hair. My chest tightened up at the thought of what my husband, James, would say when he looked at the credit card bill, but what could I do? I couldn't very well leave her to freeze.

'It's a tough one isn't it?' grimaced Danny as if reading my mind. 'My feller goes nuts with me about all the rugs I buy.'

My entire body was rigid from the stress of the ridiculous rug scenario as I drove home feeling as if I'd been hit on the head with a lump hammer.

What the hell just happened there? My mind went into overdrive. *Why did I not know about horse rugs? That cost a bloody fortune. Why have I bought a horse that can't grow its own winter coat?*

Calm down, said my common-sense brain.

Calm down? And Louise! She's such a bitch. Why can't I ever speak up for myself?

A red traffic light at some roadworks gave me a few minutes of time to calm down but it didn't ease the overwhelming sensation of sadness that had begun to grow in the depths of my heart. All my life I had been wishing for a horse. When I was a child, the only time I had been genuinely happy had been during my once-a-week riding lesson. We couldn't afford very much in those days and looking back, I wondered how we had been able to pay for the lessons. Every other day of the week had been miserable due to being so scared of school.

Why am I allowing Louise to make me feel like that again? I'm an adult now, this is ridiculous.

The lights changed to green and I moved off. I took a deep

breath and tried to relax but I could sense I was still clenching my jaw about the sheer responsibility of owning a horse and the worry of the soon-to-be-implemented winter rules. My heart thumped in my chest and I half expected to have a heart attack. However, when I arrived home, I discovered that Wrexford had left me a surprise gift in the kitchen, which took my mind off everything like magic.

'Why have you done a poo?' I couldn't believe it. It was only when I had to get ready for work when he did these things. Luckily my only massage client of the afternoon was Lady Alexa Heptonstall and she found the whole thing very amusing indeed.

'Oh dear!' she guffawed, as only the aristocracy can. 'It's rather pongy in here! Hahaa! Whippets can be rather difficult to housetrain but he'll get there in the end. Luckily it wasn't a wee. They're much harder to clear up aren't they?'

'Yes, he did one all over the cupboard doors this morning,' I replied.

'Oh whoops.' Alexa snorted with laughter and reminded me even more of Princess Anne.

'I can't believe how many rugs Poppy needs,' I said as we walked upstairs to my therapy room. I wouldn't normally talk about my own life with a client but Lady Alexa had been instrumental in my return to riding and she loved to hear all about my new horsey life.

'Oh yes, she will need quite a few. Were your yard mates having the "which rug?" conversation?' She chuckled knowingly.

'Yes, and I had absolutely no idea what they were talking about.'

'Oh, it's so funny. There are always several women looking at different weather apps and trying to work out which rug is best when it's going to be this or that temperature. They all end up going quite batty trying to choose which rug. I have to admit I do go a bit bonkers myself but luckily, it's just me and Tony now so not too many opinions.'

'I've never ridden a horse that needed to wear a coat before. It's completely alien to me and it cost me a fortune.' I winced at the memory of the terrible rug bill.

'Yes, there's certainly a lot to be said for cobs,' laughed Alexa.

Later that afternoon I had three seconds to breathe and calm myself before my mum brought Florence back home.

'Hello, love,' said Mum, giving me a big hug and a kiss. 'She didn't eat much dinner, did you, Florence?'

Florence looked sad, which was unlike her, and she went straight into her room to play with Wrexford.

'I think you'd better go and chat with her. She didn't have a nice time at school today.' My mum raised her eyebrows and gave me another hug, then went on her way so I could go and speak with Florence.

'Is something wrong?' I asked, sitting down on her bed. Florence nodded her head and began to speak in a wavering voice.

'Lucia stole my money for the school fair.'

'She did what?' I was stunned. Lucia was one of her best friends.

'I dropped it on the floor and she grabbed it and said "finders keepers" and she wouldn't give me it back.' Florence began to cry.

'Oh Flo! I'm so sorry to hear that happened. I'll call her mum.' I hugged her and gave her a kiss.

'No!'

'What do you mean no?' I was surprised.

'I don't want any trouble,' replied Florence.

'We can't ignore this, it's stealing!'

'I don't want you to call her mum. Please don't!'

'Well I won't if you don't want me to but we can't let this happen again,' I said firmly.

I went to the kitchen and made a cup of tea, my heart racing. I didn't want Florence to be how I had been. I needed to help her to speak up for herself. How though? What would have helped me? I had no idea. The only thing that had helped me to feel better at the time was my weekly riding lesson on a Saturday. It was the only time when my mind was free from all thoughts. All that existed was the smell of the pony and the enjoyment of grooming soft fur. I remembered the cobbled yard with the odd bit of straw strewn in the gutter that ran around the edge. The happy sound of children's chatter and the dash to the tack room to collect saddle and bridle.

'Who are you riding today?' someone would invariably shout over to a friend. I was always so happy to be there I didn't care which pony I had. I loved them all and can remember their names and quirky habits to this day.

The riding school where Florence was learning was not as lovely as my own childhood riding schools had been, so maybe it would help to find a better place and perhaps she could have two lessons a week instead. That could help to ease her mind.

Chapter 2

The week passed in a blur of the usual monotonous chores. Jack hadn't mentioned her field idea again so I assumed she'd forgotten all about it. In a way I was relieved. Although the livery yard was like being back at school again with so many different types of people to cope with, some bossy and some bitchy, it felt like a safer place to learn how to be a horse owner rather than a horse loaner. Poppy and I had been doing well as a partnership during the time I had her on loan but for some unknown reason, since I had become her owner, her behaviour had begun to be erratic again and I felt out of my depths once more. I had a rare day of no work so I decided to try to do something to help make things better. I jumped in the car and as usual, the eternal guilt set in immediately.

I should invite my mum to come with. I never make enough time to see her and she loves horses. But then I won't be able to focus on Poppy. What should I do? Oh heck.

By the time my mind had finished going round in circles I discovered I'd actually arrived at the livery yard so it was too late to call my mum. I pushed the guilt to the back of my mind and focussed on Poppy.

'Why are you so changeable?' I asked her as I managed to dodge a nip. She seemed to get cross each time I attempted to groom her right side. I reached out to try again. She snorted and did a tap dance, kicking her grooming tools across the floor of the barn. She stared at me with wide eyes and flared her already large nostrils. 'I thought you'd got over all this,' I sighed as I went to gather them up. 'If you stay like this, it's going to be a miserable situation for both of us.'

Poppy swung her rump round and knocked me sideways onto the cold, hard floor. My elbow stung. My enthusiasm instantly disappeared and I lost all desire to take her into the school so instead, I led her back to the field, turned her loose and watched her prance off into the distance.

Why did I do that? I was annoyed with myself. *I should have tried some connection work. It's not going to get better if I don't try.* I walked back to the barn and tidied up, which helped me to ignore my thoughts.

'Great, you're here!' said Jack as she strode through the massive barn doors, looking around to check we were alone. 'I've made a list of where we should look for land.' She passed me a crumpled paper bag on which she had scrawled a list of notes. My heart sank as I had hoped she had forgotten all about it, but I mustered up some fake enthusiasm and had a look at her list. It made no sense whatsoever.

'Mad woman's field near the garden centre?' I read out loud. 'Where the heck's that? And what's "creepy mansion near Valerie's back garden is big enough for horses"? I doubt Valerie would let us keep our horses in her back garden. Is it really that big?' Valerie was the owner of the livery yard where I had first met Jack when I was loaning a pony there.

'No! It's a creepy-looking mansion on the road *near* Valerie's yard. The back garden is absolutely massive! We should give it a go and see if we can get it.'

'I don't like the sound of being at a creepy mansion. What if it's haunted?' I was very wary.

'Don't be daft,' laughed Jack. 'You're bloody nuts you are!'

'Well what's the mad woman's field near the garden centre?' I felt quite concerned about that place too.

'You know the one? It's completely hidden by forty-foot hedges and you can't see it at all. Everyone says the woman who owns it is a total lunatic.'

'Well no I definitely haven't seen a field that's hidden by giant hedges,' I laughed. 'And do we really want to rent some land from a mad woman?'

'She might not be that bad? I'll show you it. You'll love it.'

Jack drove at break-neck speed towards the village. Her van was full of empty cans of cola and screwed up paper bags from the bakery which flew around my feet as she screeched round the corners. It certainly made me feel a whole lot better about my own filthy car, which was almost pristine in comparison.

The hidden field was near the garden centre and to get in we had to climb over a rusty old gate into a very derelict-looking small, paved yard. It was overgrown with ancient weeds that had taken quite a hold, but around a corner it opened out into something else entirely.

'Oh … my… God,' I gasped. 'Wow!'

'It's amazing, isn't it?' Jack looked around and smiled.

'It's like walking into a fairy tale.' I couldn't believe what I was seeing. 'The grass is so green and thick! And look at that enormous oak tree in the middle, it must be hundreds of years old.'

'My favourite's the willow tree over there by the stream.' Jack pointed to the most majestic willow, its long tendrils tickling the top of the water and waving slightly in the breeze.

'Wow yes, that's a beautiful stream. It's so wide, the horses would love it. How big is this place? It looks absolutely massive.'

'I think it's about ten acres,' Jack replied.

'It's like something out of a film set. I just can't get over how vivid the colours are and it's so enormous yet completely hidden. I wonder how it's not completely overgrown with weeds?' I looked up at the mountainous hedgerow in awe. Nature clearly loved the place as there were many different types of birds singing the most beautiful songs and iridescent dragon flies swooping through the air. It was peculiar to see them this late in the season but the place was so sheltered it almost had its own micro climate.

'Look at that,' I gasped. 'I've never seen a heron in real life. Oh it's caught a fish!'

We stood there for some time, watching the ethereal heron wading in the stream, transfixed by the unadulterated beauty of the whole place. It looked so pure and untouched by humans that we daren't walk further in and sully it.

'Oi!' shouted an unfriendly voice, which made us both jump. 'What the hell do you think you're doing here?' A rather large, military-looking old lady, wearing a grubby green tweed coat and beige breeches, was marching towards us. Her thick, grey frizzy hair bounced with each step.

'What are you doing on my land?' she demanded, her eyes looking in two different directions at once. 'I've a bloody good mind to call the police!'

'Oh heck. Sorry,' I blurted anxiously. 'We were just having a look. We were hoping to be able to rent it for our horses. Would that be possible?' Jack seemed to be frozen from the shock of meeting the infamous 'mad woman'.

'No it would definitely not be blasted possible! The cheek of it. Trespassing on my land and then as bold as brass asking if you can bring your horses here? To blazes with the pair of you. Get off my land before I call the constabulary!'

By now Jack's mouth had dropped open and my face had gone bright red. I had no idea how to reply to the woman, mainly because she sounded like someone out of an Enid Blyton book, but also she had the most deranged expression on her face that I thought she might actually try to kill us or something.

'Er, ok I am so sorry,' I managed to mumble as I grabbed Jack's arm and we both dashed away.

'Bloody hell,' snorted Jack as she exploded into laughter from the safety of her van. 'What the hell just happened then?'

'I think that was the mad woman that you mentioned earlier,' I replied, fanning my hot face with a handy magazine that I found in the footwell. 'If she'd had a shotgun she would have killed us.'

'God yes. She was terrifying! Let's get out of here.'

'Yes let's,' I agreed and we sped off down the lane.

Jack pulled into a layby a safe distance away. 'Well, I think we can strike that off the list.'

'What a shame though. It looked perfect. I could have lived there myself, never mind the horses,' I sighed.

'Yeah me too. It's the most stunning place I've ever see. I knew you'd love it. Oh well, what's next on the list?'

'The creepy mansion.' I grimaced. 'Not liking the sound of this.'

'Oh yes, it's not far from here.' Jack glanced in her mirrors and set off.

The creepy mansion looked like something from *The Munsters*. It was the last property on a very weird, perfectly straight road that featured several ridiculously enormous houses. I say houses in the loosest sense of the word because they were really palaces or were they prisons? They may as well have been for all the security fences, gates, cameras and personal guards on patrol.

'Could you live here?' I asked Jack.

'No! Are you mental? I can only just afford the council house I rent,' she laughed.

'I mean, if you were a millionaire would you live here?'

'Oh right, I see what you mean. No chance,' she replied, shaking her head. 'It's like a posh jail, isn't it?'

'Yes, that's exactly what I was thinking.'

We both stepped out onto the street and the private security guards drove straight over to let us know we had been *noticed*. We smiled and waved. They observed us, stony faced, and then drove slowly past and parked up nearby.

'What a boring job that must be,' laughed Jack as we made our way to the gates of the creepy mansion. The gates were open and the long driveway was full of building rubble, old wooden beams and a few massive skips overflowing with rubbish.

'Hello ladies! Can I help you?' greeted a scruffy-looking man with a thick cockney accent, pushing a wheelbarrow full of broken bricks. He reached up to scratch his shiny bald head, emitting an acrid smell of BO which burned the back of my throat. I was fascinated by his bristly neck and couldn't quite work out what the blurred tattoo was meant to be. It looked sort of like a devil, or perhaps a pig, it was hard to tell.

'Hi, we're looking for the owner,' said Jack.

'Well you've found him.' The man grinned and revealed a gold tooth that actually glinted in the sunlight. All that was missing was a high-pitched 'ping' and it would have been perfect.

'Oh!' we both must have looked very surprised so the man explained he had recently bought the house and was renovating it.

'Right,' nodded Jack. 'Looks like a big job. We were just wondering if you might consider renting us some of your back garden for our horses?'

The man looked over at the garden as if he'd only just realised it was there.

'Yeah, hmm, now that's a good point,' the man scratched his head. 'It's massive isn't it? We will need something doing with that won't we? I definitely don't want to mow it, haha! Are you two quite experienced with horses then?'

'Yes, we've had them for years,' Jack replied with great confidence.

'Speak for yourself,' I muttered under my breath, wondering why he would ask that question.

'I'll tell you what. You can bring your horses here and then in return you can teach my kids to ride. How about that? I'll build you a stable yard too,' the man walked over to the fence next to the field/garden and had a good look round.

'We can't teach kids how to ride,' I hissed at Jack.

'Shhh! Yes we can!' she whispered back. I felt a bit sick at the thought of it. I did not have the time or the knowledge to teach some random blokes' kids how to ride.

'I don't know when it'll be ready 'cos I need to get the house sorted first and as you can see it's a big job. Come and have a look round.'

I didn't want to go inside the house but the man had a peculiar magnetic aura about him and we found ourselves inextricably pulled into the creepy mansion.

'The old feller who lived here before was found dead on the stairs,' laughed our host, gesturing to the wide, sweeping staircase that wound up and round to a circular gallery with many doors leading to God only knew where. 'He'd been dead for about four months, so they say, so there weren't much left of 'im!'

'Jeez,' Jack remarked.

'Yeah it took ages to clean his body off the wood. Ha! Glad I didn't have to do that. Can you imagine the smell? Well anyway, I'm going to get the whole place sorted out and keep the original features,' he pointed to some beautiful scrollwork on the banisters. 'And me and the wife'll host some special parties if you know what I mean?' he winked and smirked. It made me feel very uneasy.

'Now this is my favourite room.' He led us into a very dark drawing room filled with moth-eaten velvet-covered furniture that had seen better days. 'I reckon I'll turn this room into the dungeon hahaa! I know what you ladies like.' The man grinned, revealing his gold tooth once again. Jack and I were too shocked to reply so we just smiled dumbly.

'The wife was a pole dancer at one of my clubs and she's big into swinging. Maybe you ladies would like to join us? We like a bit of fresh meat.' He threw his head back and laughed almost hysterically. I felt my heart pause for a disturbingly long time and I wanted to vomit.

Luckily, the weird man led us back outside into the light, which was a huge relief as I thought our end had come.

'Anyway, ladies, there's a lot to do, plus I've got a new nightclub that needs refurbing but give me your phone numbers and I'll call you when it's ready,' said the man as we walked back up the driveway.

I didn't want to give him my phone number because he made me feel very uneasy but I felt that I had no option. So I gave him a few wrong digits instead. Just as he was typing it into his phone, a sleek, black car rolled up and a group of very large men got out and leered at us. The hairs on the back of my neck stood on end and I wanted to run away very fast. Fortunately, fate intervened and the man's phone rang so we were able to make a hasty exit.

'Jesus Christ,' I gasped as we got into Jack's van. 'I thought we were going to get murdered – again.'

'Yeah he was a bit scary wasn't he? Did you see his neck tat?' she laughed.

'Yes! And his gold tooth!'

'I don't want to go to their freaky parties,' said Jack with a shiver.

'Me neither.' I shook my head. 'I can't believe what weirdos we've met and we're only looking for a field to rent.'

Jack smiled and waved at the weird men as we drove away and eventually pulled into the layby opposite Valerie's ramshackle yard.

'I do miss being here,' she sighed wistfully. 'We had fun didn't we?'

'Yes,' I agreed. 'I still wish I'd bought Monty.'

'Do you really?' asked Jack, surprised. 'He was so slow.'

'He was slow, yes, but I had such a deep bond with him. And he could grow his own coat and didn't need shoes. I just hope he's in a good home now.'

'Yes, I hope so too,' Jack nodded.

We sat in silence for a while, enjoying the view and our memories and we munched on a large bag of crisps.

'Let's get out and have a walk,' said Jack when we had finished eating. 'I just want to check something out.'

'Ok,' I said as we stepped out of the van. Jack headed straight for the bridle path that ran along the edge of the 'abandoned field' next to Valerie's yard. This was the field that drove Valerie crazy on a regular basis due to the abundance of weed seeds that blew into her pristine fields.

'There must be a way in somewhere,' Jack muttered poking through the overgrown hedges.

'You're not thinking of renting this field are you?' I was aghast. 'It's like a jungle! And we would have Valerie as our next-door neighbour and you know where that will lead.'

'What do you mean?' asked Jack, bemused.

'She'll expect you to look after her donkeys again.'

'Oh heck the dreaded donkeys. I'm not doing that,' laughed Jack. 'Ooh look! It's a gate!'

Jack had found the gate into the mysterious field. It was ancient and rusty, covered in a thick tangle of brambles and tied closed to a post with a thin chain and muddy padlock.

'Let's go in,' said Jack excitedly as she climbed over the gate. 'Ouch! Bloody prickles. My foot! Aaarghh!' Jack's boot had somehow got stuck in the gate, which made her lose her balance. She sailed over the gate in an extremely haphazard way and landed with a resounding thud into the undergrowth. 'Ow bollocks.'

'Oh God. Are you ok?' I called out.

'I'll live,' she groaned, as she scrambled to her feet. I climbed over the gate as carefully as I could but still managed to rip my jeans on the brambles.

'Wow,' I whistled. 'This is like that film, *Jumanji*.' I had never seen a field that had become so overgrown. The tall grasses and thistles almost reached my waist and many other weeds had grown so tall some of them were at eye level. It was almost impossible to walk around in it. It was a good workout as we had to lift our legs really high to get anywhere.

'Where the heck are we now?' I exclaimed as it dawned on me I couldn't see anything except grass and giant weeds.

'I think we're heading in the direction of Valerie's? Or are we going towards the golf course? I have no idea,' Jack laughed her head off. 'Let's get out of here! This was a bad idea.'

After what felt like an eternity of battling with nature we finally found our way to the gate again.

'Crikey, I'm knackered,' I gasped as I climbed out of the field, relieved to be back on the bridle path.

'It's such a waste of a good field though isn't it?' Jack shook her head. 'Ah well, let's call it a day. We can look again another time.'

Jack dropped me back at the yard and I noticed I still had time to do something with Poppy before home life needed me back. I walked with purpose into the barn to collect her headcollar and strode nonchalantly to the field. My heart sank as I noticed Louise was turning her horse loose but I wasn't going to let her see I was rattled.

'Poppy!' I called. Poppy looked up and then a passing wagon, honking its horn, spooked her and she galloped off round the field. None of the other horses bothered to join in her mad reaction.

'I really don't know why you think she'd come to call,' said Louise. 'A horse like that needs an experienced owner and let's face it, that isn't you, is it? You're far too soft with her. She'd respect you more if you used a firmer hand.' She gave a tinkly laugh and walked away.

I steadied myself on the fence and took a deep breath. I felt like I'd been hit by a force ten gale.

What an absolutely horrible cow! I spluttered inwardly.

Poppy walked over and stood near me, just watching. Then she lowered her head to be closer to me. I could tell she sensed I wasn't ok and her presence was something of a comfort. It was a relief that there was still a connection between us despite the nastiness of Louise's words. I leaned into her and took a gulp of air. The scent of her body took me right back to my riding lessons. How I relished the smell of the ponies and how I loved to just stand with them in the stable after the lesson, wishing that moment could last forever.

'You can have two riding lessons a week if it will help you to feel better,' I remembered my mum saying. I must have been about fourteen when I finally reached the point where life had become too much to deal with.

But I am an adult now, I reasoned with myself. *I don't need to feel this crap just because that awful woman always says nasty things. Come on, Grace, get a grip.*

I waited with Poppy for as long as I could and then headed back towards my car, relieved to find that Louise had already left.

I know, I'll book a riding lesson with Elise. I am not going to let that evil cow make me feel like death again.

I took a deep breath and called my riding instructor. I felt a lot better knowing that I had done something practical to help myself and Poppy.

Chapter 3

Knowing I had a riding lesson gave me the boost I needed to set off to the livery yard with a positive attitude. I was surprised to see so many cars in the carpark when I arrived as usually no one was there at lunchtime on a Wednesday.

'I told you that horse would be the death of you!' June's daughter was fuming with rage as she marched out of the barn and strode towards her car. June was sitting in her wheelchair inside, drinking a cup of very sweet tea with a shaky hand.

'Oh no! What happened?' I asked, looking at everyone's glum expressions.

'Beatrix has been up to her old tricks again,' sighed Sally. 'She reared and almost had June off this time and she was only walking round the school.'

'That's weird. I wonder why? Did you ever book a lesson with Elise?' I asked.

'No but that's a very good idea,' nodded June, her ginger curls bouncing as her head moved.

'Do you think that's wise dear?' asked her husband, David, tentatively, clasping and unclasping his hands.

'Well what else can I do?' June replied with wide eyes.

'Er, well er maybe you could perhaps, ahem, er you know, er, sell her?' suggested David, his face growing red as he pulled on the sleeves of his knitted, beige cardigan.

'Sell her? David! I can't believe you could even think that. Beatrix is my dream come true! I am not giving up just because she likes to stand on end!'

I couldn't believe my ears. I didn't even have a terrible back problem like June yet I would absolutely not dare to sit on a horse that reared.

'Grace, give me Elise's number. I am going to call her now.' June folded her arms defiantly. David sighed in his usual resigned manner, his care-worn face lined with worry. He muttered something incoherent and took his glasses off to clean them.

I felt very uncomfortable and tried not to look at David as I gave June Elise's number and wandered off to get Poppy, eventually realising that the reason why I was going to get Poppy was because I actually had a lesson booked with Elise. I laughed at myself and then managed to stumble into the electric fence.

'Ow!' I leaped into the air from the shock. 'God, can I get any more stupid today?'

'Probably! You can be quite daft can't you?' replied Jack cheerfully. She was turning Buddy into the field. 'What do you think about June?'

'I think she's either super brave or extremely mad. What do you think?'

'I think she's mad. I wouldn't ride that horse even without a history of back problems like hers. There's something not right with it. She could end up paralysed if she comes off and she's only just getting her walking back,' Jack sighed. 'But it's her choice.'

'Well maybe Elise can talk some sense into her?' I wondered.

'Doubt it.' Jack shook her head. 'June is too stubborn.'

When we arrived back at the barn, Elise had arrived and was listening to the sorry tale of Beatrix and her weird rearing. Elise was a very no-nonsense ex-racehorse trainer and as usual she was wearing her smart tweed jacket and dark corduroy trousers. I could feel my body begin to relax just by being near her due to her positive nature.

'Have you spoken to the previous owner?' asked Elise. 'They might be able to shed some light on this behaviour.' As ever, Elise's sensible mind went immediately to the possible cause of the problem.

'Oh! No I hadn't thought of that,' June replied. 'She was from a dealer so I'm not sure if he would know much about it.'

'It's still worth asking,' suggested Elise.

'Yes, ok. I'll do that now.' June opened her phone and called the dealer while I went into Poppy's stable to get her ready for her lesson.

'Right, Grace, let's get going!' said Elise briskly when Poppy was tacked up, and she marched us off to the school.

'Walk her around in-hand first!' she called out as I led Poppy through the gate. 'Let's see how she's moving!' Elise was the sort of enthusiastic person who sounded as if every sentence ended with an exclamation mark.

I walked Poppy round the whole perimeter of the school, smiling with the relief of being once again in the capable presence of my riding instructor.

'It's important to do a body check before we ride and it's time you learned how to do it yourself!' called Elise from the centre of the school where she was standing with her hands on her hips, studiously watching Poppy with her eagle eyes.

'A body check?' I repeated.

'Yes! Bring her into the centre … aaaand halt!'

'What's a body check?' I asked.

'Each time you've had a lesson, have you noticed that I run my hands over her while you're grooming and tacking up?'

'Er, not really no.' I hadn't noticed any of that.

'Good! That means I've become a ninja body tester,' laughed Elise. 'I didn't want to overload you before because there was never anything wrong but now that she's your horse it's vital to understand the main causes of so-called *bad behaviour*.'

'Great,' I nodded. 'This sounds interesting.'

'Yes, it is interesting and as you do massage I think you'll find it easy to understand. Now take her saddle off and just prop it by the fence.'

I followed the instructions and hurried back to Poppy, full of zeal.

'Ok, so here we have a horse. Now get down on all fours so you can get an idea of how it feels to actually be a horse.'

'Pardon?' I laughed. I thought she was joking.

'Yes, seriously! Just for a moment.'

With some reservations, I got down on all fours.

'Now obviously your body is not the same as a horse but see how it feels when I push down on your back,' said Elise as she pressed her hand onto my back and put a bit of weight through it.

'Oh yikes! That's a bit weird! I don't like that!'

'Exactly. Ok you can stand up now,' she chuckled. 'Even though the horse has four legs, their spine is still the same basic idea as ours. Now, we have our head at the top of our body and the weight travels down our back comfortably because the spine is stacked vertically. Imagine having to carry that head weight all day if your back was horizontal? You would need a very strong core to compensate for that wouldn't you?'

'I'd never thought about it,' I replied. 'But yes, you're right.'

'The back of a horse is not designed to carry a rider. Think of all that weight pushing down on a small section of the spine. Unless the abdominal muscles are strong and the neck muscles are relaxed, trouble will be brewing. The saddle is designed to spread the weight but if it doesn't fit correctly, it can cause other problems.'

I mulled over what she was saying.

'Now we know your saddle fits correctly. But even so, it's vital to do regular pole work – it strengthens the tummy muscles. That then protects the back. So, have a feel all the way down her back and watch to see if she reacts to your touch,' Elise instructed.

I ran my hand down Poppy's back from her withers to her bum. Her shoulder muscles fluttered as we went over them.

'Now that's very subtle but it's showing you she has a bit of sensitivity and I would guess it's her neck that's causing that.'

'Really? Why?' I was fascinated.

'It's the way she holds her head with tension. She just needs to learn to relax and then that will help her shoulders. It's nothing serious, but it could become serious if you don't nip it in the bud now.'

'Oh heck. How do I do that?' Panic began to rise in my chest.

'Give her a massage every now and then,' suggested Elise. 'It will help her to feel closer to you, which might help improve her behaviour. And relax yourself. If it gets worse, she'll need a physio session. Sports horses nearly always end up with problems! And I wouldn't be surprised if Poppy does end up needing a physio because she does have a back that's quite long and her head is a bit oversized.'

'Oh hell, more expense.'

'Yes, I'm afraid it's a bit like the difference between a Fiat Panda and a Porsche. Sports cars have more that can go wrong!' Elise laughed cheerfully as if it was a joke. I wasn't amused. I could feel a tightness in my chest at the thought of having bought this type of horse and Louise's searing remarks wormed their way into my mind.

'The main thing is, you're aware of it,' said Elise matter-of-factly. 'So you can do everything with more care and hopefully avoid a big vet bill! Now let's move on to other parts of her body.'

Elise prodded various bits of Poppy, including her legs, chest and back end, to show me how to check for any possible soreness. It was very quick and luckily there were no reactions so Poppy was fine to ride.

'It's important to do this regularly so that you can rule out any pain-related behaviour issues. Right, now let's saddle up and on you get and walk her around the whole school in both directions. The more you get her mind working the better she will be for you!'

Oh my God now she needs a physio. I worried silently in my head.

Not necessarily if you do things carefully, replied my sensible side.

Yes she will! Her back's too long! Why is her back too long? And her head's too big! Bloody hell. Why have I bought this type of horse?

The lesson passed in a blur. My mind was so busy worrying about Poppy potentially ending up with a back problem that I barely took any notice of what we were doing.

'Right! That's enough for today, you aren't fully here anyway. I can hear your mind worrying,' Elise laughed heartily. 'Don't overthink it. Just take it one day at a time!'

'Hmmm, I'll try.' I screwed my face up, sighed deeply and

dismounted. Poppy put her nose on my cheek as if to apologise and that made me feel a wave of guilt. 'I do love you,' I said to her and gave her a kiss.

'In time it will all feel more normal. It's just an adjustment. It's a big thing to go from loaning cobs to buying a sports horse.' Elise winked. 'Now let's see what this Beatrix has to offer us!'

Beautifully timed, Beatrix and June appeared in the distance being chaperoned by Jack, Sally and Alex, who had just arrived and wanted to watch what Elise would do. Beautiful Beatrix, her silver dapples shining in the autumn sun, walked very calmly next to the wheelchair and appeared to be the perfect horse for June.

'Right! Bring her in and let the circus begin!' called Elise cheerily. Nothing ever seemed to phase her, it was as if she'd seen it all before many times.

'Did you manage to get hold of the dealer?' she asked.

'No, funnily enough the number didn't work any more,' replied June.

'Oh dear. Well that's not unheard of. Never mind, let's make the best of it. Ok, who can walk her in-hand so I can see how she moves?' asked Elise.

'I'll do it!' said Alex, who loved to help.

'Jolly good, just walk her with a long rein so we can see what she does with her head. And may I say I do like your green hair! It's very unusual!'

'Thanks!' grinned Alex. 'I like to be different.'

'You're not kidding,' sniggered Jack.

Alex walked Beatrix round the school in both directions and nothing seemed in any way wrong.

'Now we will do the body check I just taught Grace,' said

Elise, removing Beatrix's saddle. She expertly ran her hand along her back, round her bottom, under her girth, over her chest, up and down her neck and all of her legs.

'Well that's all in order. Let's check her teeth and gums.' We all held our breath, knowing how bitey Beatrix could be, but she was absolutely angelic and her mouth was fine.

'Ok, let's see if her expression changes when we put the saddle back on,' said Elise, inviting Sally to put the saddle on. 'If the saddle is uncomfortable, Beatrix will let us know – hopefully! Most horses do at any rate.' Sally put the saddle on and Beatrix remained calm and relaxed.

'Well, we have seen that there is nothing wrong physically and nothing wrong with the tack. So I will now ride her.' We all gasped.

'Good luck,' I said.

'It's ok! It's a soft landing!' laughed Elise and nonchalantly mounted.

Round and round the school she went several times in walk, trot and canter and Beatrix behaved beautifully as if butter wouldn't melt. Eventually, Elise brought her back to a halt.

'Well I have absolutely no idea why you have been hav— aaaarghhhh bloody hell!' Beatrix went up on her back legs, paddled her front legs for a second and then returned to earth and stood calmly. Elise jumped off and fanned herself.

'Crikey! How peculiar!' she said.

'That's one word for it.' Jack smirked.

'What's wrong with her?' wailed June, her eyes wide with fear.

'Do you know what I think?' said Alex, standing back with her hands on her hips, staring deeply at Beatrix.

'Oh God, here we go,' sighed Jack. 'Don't tell me, she's got the spirit of a Native American trapped up her arse and that's why she's rearing?' Everyone laughed. Alex was well known for her other-worldly view on life, which Jack never had much patience for.

'Actually no. I was not going to say that,' laughed Alex good naturedly. 'What I was going to say, before you rudely interrupted, was that I think she has been taught to do this. Her face just looks like she thinks this is what she's meant to do.'

'I suppose that's a possibility,' nodded Elise. 'She is very calm.'

'Why would anyone teach a horse to do that?' exclaimed June in a very high-pitched voice.

'Just for fun?' I offered.

'Yes, you know, now you say it, she does appear to believe that's a normal thing to do,' agreed Sally.

'Good God, it's not the sort of normal I'd want from a horse,' said Jack. 'What are you going to do, June?'

'Oh heck I don't know. I just don't know!' wailed June, wringing her hands.

'There must be a cue that causes her to do it,' I wondered out loud.

'Yes maybe,' said Elise. 'You just need to work out what it is and try to either not do it or teach her to do something else instead.'

'Yes, like keep all four feet on the ground,' said Jack, shaking her head. 'I know what I would do but it's your horse, June.'

'Oh dear oh dear!' June was very stressed.

'I'll tell you what I think you should do,' said Alex.

'Oh God,' sighed Jack.

'I think you should just learn to cope with it, like a trick rider!'

Sally roared with laughter, 'Oh Alex, you're so potty!'

'That sounds crazy!' I said.

'No! I am serious! All she does is go up in the air, wave her arms about and then she comes back down,' replied Alex.

'Her arms?' I asked.

'I mean her front legs!'

'Oh my God this is the maddest thing you've ever suggested,' said Jack. 'June will fall off backwards and break her back.'

'Not if she goes to a professional stunt rider who could teach her how to sit to it!' replied Alex emphatically.

'Now I know you've gone completely nuts,' laughed Jack, shaking her head. Her dreadlocks hit me in the eye. 'Oh, sorry Grace. Look this is the most idiotic conversation. Something serious needs to be done.'

'Hang on a minute,' Alex pulled her phone out of her pocket. 'There's a Western teacher somewhere not that far from here. I bet he could help with this. Aha! Found him.' Alex smiled smugly and showed us his homepage, which featured a photo of him on a horse that was rearing. 'Call him up. It's worth a go!'

'Oh heck, I don't know what David will think of all this,' said June.

'Like he could stop you,' muttered Jack.

'Well yes obviously he can't actually stop me, but he'll be worried to death.'

'I'll call him! It looks so exciting, I want to learn how to ride like this,' said Alex, dialling the number. 'Ooh we should all go! Won't that be fun?'

'No. It would be the opposite of fun,' replied Jack. 'I am going to have a nice quiet cup of tea while I've still got time before work. Good luck, June!' And with that she wandered off.

I had to go too because I had work beckoning, so I walked towards the barn with Jack.

'She'll end up in that wheelchair permanently,' I sighed. 'But what can you do? It's her choice.'

'Yes,' agreed Jack. 'As my Jamaican nan would say "Haad ears pickny nyam rockstone". She'll have to learn the hard way.'

I sighed and nodded. June was an amazingly strong-minded woman in her mid-sixties who I deeply admired and she was recovering well from her back operations to fix some bulging lumbar discs. The thought of her ruining it all just out of stubbornness really saddened me. But there was nothing anyone could say to change her opinion once she had set her mind on something. I had my own anxieties to cope with, though, and didn't have much headspace to worry about June. I led Poppy back to the field and gave her a kiss for being so well behaved in her lesson.

'If you could always be like this, that would be great,' I said, hoping that she might understand. I turned her loose and she sauntered over to a quiet part of the field to graze alone.

My therapy room was ready for the first patient of the day. I loved that room. It was at the very top of the house and full of light thanks to the large Velux window. The walls were a pale cream and all the soft furnishings were purple. It was my sanctuary and the only room in the house where I could be guaranteed peace and quiet. I took a few deep breaths, relaxed my mind and warmed my body up. Doing massage is so physical, it's like a workout.

The first person was Valentina. She was a very pretty blond Swiss woman and was very serious about health and fitness. She was always trying various diet fads and exercise regimes and she looked amazingly youthful despite being almost twenty years older than me.

'Hallo! Hallo!' she greeted as she bounced through the door. 'You'll never guess where I went this morning! I'll tell you because you will not be able to wonder ...' Valentina talked ten to the dozen with tremendous effervescence. I rarely got a word in edgeways but I didn't mind, she was so fascinating and positive.

'So you must now tell me how is your horse?' she asked after telling me all about her morning's experience – a colonic irrigation. I told her about how Jack and I had been looking for land to rent but with no luck.

'Oh you should come to our field! I told you this before when you were riding the little black horse. It's still available you know. Well we do have one lady there but I tell you she is so much of a problem. Perhaps you could help?'

'A problem?' I asked. I didn't like the sound of that.

'Yes! Oh dear this girl. She has three ponies and I tell you, she has not paid any rent for seven years. Well she does occasionally when we get really mad with her but she always is crying poverty, you know what I am saying?'

'Wow! That's a bit rude,' I replied.

'Yes, so very rude. Anyway, if you and your friend bring your horses, then perhaps that will make her pay?'

'Ermm, I don't really know about that,' I laughed.

'Well why don't you come to see it tomorrow? My husband will show you around: he deals with the land. I will tell him to expect you at six p.m. yes? That is good for you?' Valentina insisted and I felt we had nothing to lose by looking, so I agreed.

Chapter 4

Valentina lived in a small village called Acer which was on the
outskirts of a very grand sprawling estate named Deerwood. The
lane that led to Valentina's house was not what I expected. Even
though I knew their address, I mistakenly thought they lived
in a spooky-looking modern farm house on the other side of the
village closer to the main road. That was one of the reasons why I
hadn't wanted to consider going to look at their field.

'This is gorgeous!' said Jack as we drove down the winding
lane and marvelled at the beautiful rolling fields all around. In
the distance, the reservoir twinkled like diamonds through the
pine woods. 'I wonder if we can ride the horses round there?
Doesn't it look like a Scottish loch? Why didn't we come here
first?'

'Because I thought they lived in that big, creepy farmhouse
near the dog kennels,' I replied. 'I don't know why because I know
their address.'

'You blithering idiot! Oh well never mind, we're here now. I
wonder what her husband's like.' We didn't have to wonder for
long as a brand-new silver Bentley pulled into the drive just as we
arrived. The door swung open and the driver leaped out as if he'd
been stung by a wasp.

'Bloody fuck,' he greeted with a voice reminiscent of Michael
Caine. 'You must be Grace and Jack?' He looked us up and down,
disapprovingly. 'Well come on, I'm a busy man.' He marched off
towards his garden fence without introducing himself and I had
forgotten his name so I felt very awkward.

'He's got a ponytail,' hissed Jack. 'He looks like Mick Hucknall dressed for a wedding.'

'Shhh!' I hissed back. 'He'll hear us.' He did look very similar to Mick Hucknall though, except more muscular like a bodybuilder and he was wearing a very smart navy-blue suit that looked like it cost thousands of pounds.

'Hurry up!' he called, with great exasperation. 'Bloody gate is stuck.' He gave it a kick and it fell open. It looked like it was a hundred years old and about to completely disintegrate.

The ancient gate led into a very unkempt, overgrown field that had huge banks of nettles and giant thistles all over the place. Three horses – well, one small horse and two ponies – eyed us with suspicion. Out of nowhere a big, brindle Boxer dog bounded over to greet us.

'Bugsy! How did you get out? He's always getting out, this dog.'

Bugsy gave us both a sniff and ran off to greet the horses, suddenly letting out a loud yelp as one of them kicked him in the head.

'Those bastard horses are a menace!' shrieked Valentina's husband as he sped over to his dog and yelled obscenities to the horses, who had galloped off anyway. Jack raised her eyebrows and I felt increasingly uncomfortable. Luckily the horses were barefoot so the dog was fine, but the man was extremely cross.

'I'm bloody sick to the back teeth of that woman. She's had her horses here for seven years and hardly paid a penny. Seven fucking years! She must think I'm a soft touch. Well I suppose I am, aren't I? Anyway, you can bring your horses here if you sort that woman out. Tell her she either has to pay rent or leave. I don't want to see you or hear you so don't be bringing all your friends here, ok? I like my privacy. And don't ask me to pay for anything because I'm not interested. The weeds, the fences, I don't give a shit.' And with that he marched back through the old gate, across his garden and into his house without saying another word to us.

'Jeez, what's his problem?' whistled Jack looking at the house, which was an enormous and beautiful, old stone farmhouse covered in ivy.

'I have absolutely no idea,' I laughed, through shock more than amusement.

'Shall we walk round the field?'

'I don't know. Shall we?'

'Might as well?' suggested Jack.

We tiptoed back into the field and walked all around. It was wild and undulating and almost split into two long strips by a very old line of hawthorn that was probably meant to be a hedge but hadn't been maintained so there were lots of gaps that the horses could get through.

'It's very beautiful here,' I conceded, taking in the views of the pine woods at the bottom left of the field. The blue of the reservoir shimmered through the trees and made me wish I could go and swim in it.

'Yes,' agreed Jack, 'it really is very beautiful. Except for the drystone wall at the top there. Looks like it's about to collapse and all the fencing is about a million years old. But even so, I love how the farmland seems to go on forever all around. I can't believe how countryside it is yet we're only five minutes from suburbia. I want to move the horses here. Do you?'

No! It's too much responsibility! This is too stressful! shrieked my mind.

But it's the perfect opportunity to get away from Louise…

'Yes,' I nodded. *Shit. Why did I say yes?*

'Brilliant!' Jack whooped. 'We'll have to fill in all the gaps in this hedge line so that we can have one field resting while they graze the other. It'll be a big job but we can do it. Not sure about him, though. He's a scary bugger, isn't he?' said Jack.

'Yes and I can't remember his name. I think it might be Roger?' I wondered. 'He really is a very scary guy.' *He's seriously scary! Why have I agreed to this madness? I'm going to be sick.*

'We'll just have to keep out of his way and be as quiet as possible. How much is the rent? He never said, did he?'

'No he didn't. I'll ask Valentina, and I'll ask her what his name is.' I sent her a quick text.

'What's she like?' asked Jack.

'Absolutely lovely and she's stunning too. You'll probably fancy her,' I laughed.

'Well that's something to look forward to. Shame she's married to that weirdo. Oh God here comes his dog again.' Jack bent down to greet Bugsy, who jumped all over her and then shot through the hedge out onto the lane.

'Oh for God's sake.' Jack jumped up. 'We'd better go and get him before he gets runover. We'll get the blame from what's-his-name if he does.' We both dashed over to the gate that led to the road. It wouldn't open so we had to climb over it.

'Where did he go?' I wondered out loud.

'He's over there!' Jack spotted him further down the lane. 'Bugsy!' she called out.

Bugsy wagged his tail and ran off at top speed. We both automatically ran after him, puffing and panting. He eventually led us to a pub round the corner. He jumped at the door, pushed it open and went inside.

'Your usual, Bugsy?' we heard the barman say as we both hurtled through the door, exhausted from the chase.

'Bloody hell,' spluttered Jack as she almost fell to her knees by the bar.

'Hello, ladies. Are you alright? Do you need an ambulance?' The jolly-looking barman smirked.

'That bloody dog,' I gasped.

'Bugsy? He always comes in here. He's a regular,' laughed the man. 'Were you trying to take him home?'

'Yes,' I managed to reply. 'I'm so unfit!'

The barman poured us both a glass of fresh orange juice and laughed at us again. 'Bugsy lives round the corner. He comes in here all the time and we don't bother calling his owner any more. He goes home when he's ready.'

'Oh how crazy,' I replied. 'We're bringing our horses to their field and we thought we should rescue his dog.'

'I wouldn't bother. He'll be alright here and he'll go home later, don't worry.' The barman wandered off to serve someone else.

Jack and I sat down at a table to have our drinks and Bugsy came and lay down next to us.

'Yet another weird situation,' sighed Jack, stroking Bugsy's head. 'So what to do about this field?'

'I'll see if Valentina has replied.' I fished around in my pocket for my phone. 'Yes! She says "My husband is called Roger. £100 a month between you." Wow that's so cheap. "Please sort out the other horses." I wonder what that means?'

'God knows. Do they think we can make her pay? We don't even know her name.'

'Good point, I'll ask her.' I sent a reply to Valentina, who immediately responded. 'She says she's called Anna and they don't know her surname, but she's a dog walker apparently.'

'Right. Anna the dog walker, that's helpful,' said Jack sarcastically.

'Do you know what? I think I know her.' Something niggled in the back of my mind. A memory was trying to push forwards but I couldn't quite grab it.

'Seriously?' asked Jack incredulously.

'Yes. God what the hell am I trying to remember?' I stared at my glass while my subconscious mind worked furiously trying to piece together bits of information. 'I know the name "Anna the dog walker" and for some bizarre reason it's linked to ponies. Damn it, what is it? Who is she? Why do I know her?'

Jack bit her lip, stopping herself from interrupting my thoughts.

'Ah yes! That's it!'

'No way. What?' laughed Jack.

'I met her in Roundhay Park ages ago because she was with my friend's aunty. She's a dog walker and she was talking about these ponies her grandma had given her and she was looking for someone small to help back them and she asked me if I rode.' I sat back and grinned with relief. My brain had not let me down. 'I know it's her because she said they were near the Deerwood stately home.'

'Wow,' laughed Jack, impressed. 'It's like the end bit of *Murder She Wrote* except it's not a murder.'

'I remember feeling that I didn't want to have anything to do with the woman so I said I was too busy. She had a really dark vibe and I don't know why but when I got home I had an awful headache and I honestly felt it was from being near her.'

'Really? How weird. And how annoying that we have to deal with her. Have you got her phone number?'

'No, why?'

'We're going to have to tell her that we're coming on the field and she's going to have to pay rent,' said Jack matter-of-factly. 'There's no way I'm putting up with someone not paying their share.'

'Hmm yes. I think Valentina should do that don't you?'

'Yeah maybe,' nodded Jack. I texted Valentina, who replied saying she would tell Anna we were bringing our horses to the field and she gave me Anna's number.

'Should I message her too?' I asked.

'Yeah, it can't harm. She needs to know from the start that she has to pay. I can't believe Roger has let this go on for seven years. He seems so tough, why would he put up with it?'

'Maybe it's a front? Maybe he's really a big softie?'

'Hmmm. We'll soon find out I'm sure.' Jack shrugged her shoulders.

'Right I'll text her now. "Hi Anna, we are bringing two horses onto Valentina's field. She said she will contact you about this. So we will split the £100 rent between the three of us." What do you think?' I showed Jack the text.

'That's a good start. Add our names though.'

I included our names and sent the text. She replied instantly.

'She's replied already!'

'Read it out then,' laughed Jack.

'Oh heck she says, "I'm not very happy about this. I've had this field to myself for many years. I will be speaking with Valentina." Good luck with that, Anna.'

'Ha! Yeah! You should have paid your rent, you daft cow. I wonder what will happen next?'

My phone pinged. 'It's Valentina!'

'What's she saying? God this is stressful.'

'She said, "Anna is furious! She should have paid her rent. Do not bother with her if she gets mad with you. Bring your horses whenever you are ready, the offer is always available." Well that's good.' I put my phone back in my pocket.

'I get the feeling that they want us to evict her or make her feel so uncomfortable that she decides to leave,' said Jack.

'Yes, I think you're right. How annoying that we've got the use of this beautiful field but it comes with three ponies and a weird woman. But how amazing that it's so incredibly cheap. That will make James's day!'

'I know,' agreed Jack. 'Financially it's going to be a huge relief. I can do without the drama though, but let's just take it a day at a time. We need to plan when to move on.'

'I suppose soon, before winter?' I suggested.

'Hmm we could try. It's forecast for mild weather for the next few weeks so I'll need to build the shelter before it gets bad again. Can you ask if they'll be ok with that?'

I pulled my phone out and texted Valentina. Fortunately, she said yes so long as it was far away from the house so they couldn't see it.

'Awesome.' Jack smiled. 'I know exactly where to put it.'

We drove home and chatted excitedly about it all. Despite my initial fearful reaction, I felt relief at the fact that it was a whole world cheaper than paying livery yard fees.

'About the field shelter,' said Jack. 'I'll build it if you can pay for it.'

'Oh heck, ok.' I hadn't considered that part of it. My heart began beating fast. 'Will it cost a lot?'

'I think it'll be around two thousand. I know that sounds a lot but it would cost loads more than that to get someone else in to build it. I'll make it so that it's something we can take away if we ever have to move though, so don't worry about that.'

'Ok. I'll chat with James.' *Oh shit. He's going to go mental. What the hell have I agreed to this for?*

'It's a big outlay but in the long run it's still tons cheaper to rent land than pay livery fees.'

'Yes, I suppose so,' I nodded unconvinced. 'I'll be glad to see the back of Louise. She's become extra bitchy since I bought Poppy.'

'She's a silly cow. Probably jealous. I wouldn't bother to give her the time of day.' Jack nodded.

'I don't know why I'm letting her get to me. She makes me feel like I'm back at school.' I bit my thumb nail and stared out of the window.

'She's the classic yard bitch. Just ignore her. That's what I do.'

Ignore her. Yes I should. I wish I knew why she's suddenly making me feel so bad, my mind pondered. I felt annoyed with myself.

The day soon became early evening and I took the dinner out of the oven just as James arrived home from a busy day at the osteopathic clinic. I could see he was tired and stressed.

'I've got some news,' I ventured.

'Oh yes?' he replied, absently, looking through the day's post.

'Me and Jack have decided to move to Valentina's field.'

'Oh right. That's nice.' He scowled at the water bill.

'It's going to cost about thirty-three pounds a month.'

'What?' James looked up. 'Seriously?'

'Yes! Isn't that great?'

'That's brilliant.' He smiled. 'I know we did the right thing buying Poppy but I have to admit I was worried about the costs. When can you move on?'

'We can go whenever we like but Jack wants to build a field shelter.' My heart began booming. I coughed and swallowed. 'Jack said if we pay for it, she'll build it.'

'Oh.' James's face fell. 'And how much is that going to be?'

'Not sure,' I lied, my shoulders tightening up.

'She must have some idea?'

'Well, er, she did think it might be about, er, two thousand.' I winced.

'TWO THOUSAND POUNDS? What the hell? Why did you agree to that?'

'Because it will end up being cheaper in the long run,' I squeaked, red-faced.

'Bloody hell, Grace,' James looked away and took a deep breath.

I bit my lip and wished I could disappear, then James's phone pinged. 'Let me check this email. I'm expecting something urgent from a neurologist for a patient,' he sighed.

'Oh my God.' James looked up, shocked.

'What is it?'

'You won't believe this.' He shook his head. 'God is this true?' he read the email again. 'Yes it is.'

'What?'

'Look.' He showed me his phone.

'No way? Has that really just happened?' I was stunned.

'Yes way,' laughed James.

'I can't believe it.' I looked at the email again in case I'd misread it. But no I hadn't.

'I can't believe it either, it's like a miracle isn't it?'

'It really is a miracle. How has this just happened right now? Two thousand five hundred pounds? We've never won more than fifty quid on those savings bonds before. I'm gobsmacked.'

'Serendipity,' he laughed. 'It's all meant to be. Grace, I can see you've been stressed about buying Poppy but don't be. We can do this and I honestly feel she came into your life for a reason.' James enveloped me in a bear hug that made me cry. 'Don't cry. It's going to be ok.' Which, of course, made me cry even more.

Chapter 5

'Praise the angels for I am the absolute cleverest woman in the world!' sang green-haired Alex as I wandered into the indoor stable barn the following morning leading Poppy.

'Oh really? Why?' I laughed.

'Because I was totally right about Beatrix and the reason why she rears.' Alex smiled like a Cheshire cat.

'How do you know?'

'Because that Western guy came out last night and he rode her and said it *is* a trained habit and not a fear response.' Alex looked triumphant.

'Wow! I'm very impressed. Well done for working that out. What happens next?'

'Well that's the hard part.' Alex grimaced. 'He said she will always do it so June has to decide whether she wants to learn how to ride with it or sell her.'

'Oh blimey. What did she say?'

'As you can imagine she's not keen on the idea of selling her but neither is she keen on the idea of riding a horse that rears.'

'Oh heck, what a nightmare,' I sighed. Alex nodded her head and went to make a cup of tea.

'Hark the herald angels sing,' Veronica trilled in a terrible opera style as she swept into the barn wearing old-fashioned breeches and a hunting jacket trimmed with green velvet collar and cuffs.

'Hi Veronica,' I laughed. 'It's a bit early for Christmas carols isn't it?'

'Indeed it is! It's bonfire night soon and we must worm the horses today.' Off she went stinking of gin as usual.

'I know I'm considered to be completely potty but did any of that make any sense to you?' Alex laughed her head off.

'None at all. But do we have to worm the horses today?' I asked, a wave of anxiety washing over me.

'Oh yes. Didn't you see the notice on the board the other day? Bob wants them all treated for tapeworm before they go onto the winter field.' Alex's phone went off just at that moment so she trotted off to answer it.

I had not given any consideration to worming. Why hadn't I thought to learn about it? I felt my cheeks going red as my mind went into a spiral.

How do you worm a horse? Is it a tablet like with a dog? How would you get it in their mouth? And where is the winter field? Why don't I know any of this?

'Oh good morning, Grace. All ready for worming?' Morag strode into the barn like a ship in full sail. She was followed by Danny and Jack, who smiled and winked at me.

'Er no not really,' I admitted, my face burning hot. 'I didn't see the notice.' I felt the way I had when I was at school and everybody knew that something big was going to happen but I hadn't heard about it. It was extremely uncomfortable. Jack chuckled and went to get Buddy.

'Tch tch tch,' Morag chided, shaking her head. 'Goodness me, Grace. The notice board is a vital part of the smooth running of this community. Never mind, I have plenty of wormers so I will show you how to do it.' Morag pulled a large syringe out of her pocket and studied Poppy. 'Hmm. Now I think she probably weighs about five hundred kilos. She's a big lass isn't she?' She twiddled something on the syringe. 'We'll give her the full dose just to be sure. Right, Poppy, you will open your mouth and I don't want any nonsense.'

In one deft move, Morag grabbed Poppy in a headlock, shoved the syringe in her mouth and squirted. Poppy stood rigid, her eyes wide open like a cartoon horse. 'And do not dare to spit it out, young lady,' she commanded. There was no way Poppy was going to dare mess about with Morag.

'Right, that's you done. Does anyone else need help?' she bellowed. One after another, each horse was led over to Morag and her worming production line. All of them were extremely well behaved and took the wormer politely. 'Where are Brenda and those diabolical ponies of hers?'

'Are you going to worm them?' I asked with horror at the thought of it. 'They might kill you!'

'She's not here. She texted me to say her kids have a school concert,' said Alex.

'Well I am not going to waste my day trying to round them up,' scowled Morag. And with that she marched off to the kettle while everyone put their horses into their stables.

'Bob wants them to stay in and drop their worms before going out into the winter field,' explained Danny when he saw the confused look on my face. I felt so stupid for not knowing anything about horse worms.

'You'll get the hang of it.' He winked and wandered off.

One by one, everyone left the barn to go to work, but I had the luxury of a day off. It dawned on me that I had only ridden out on Poppy alone once and if we were considering moving to a field I needed to be able to hack on my own. My heart thumped in my chest as I began the process of grooming and tacking up, but I knew I had to do it. Luckily, she was in an amenable mood and we were soon ready to go. It was quite strange to take her to the mounting block and get on without anyone else chatting away. As I rode out of the barn I realised that I would have to go into the council estate opposite the yard, because there were a lot of roadworks going on in the village, which was further away at the back entrance of the yard. I swallowed, took a deep breath and sat tall and aimed for the main road. Poppy began to walk briskly but fortunately she stopped at the kerb so we managed to cross the road without getting killed.

'Thank God,' I said as we made it to the wide bank of grass that led into the estate. Jack had shown me a good route through the winding roads so I felt marginally confident that I could remember where we had gone. Poppy marched onwards like a war horse and my heart began to beat faster.

Calm down! commanded the sensible part of my brain. *Breathe, Grace, relax! You can do this!*

Oh my God why is she walking so fast? Is this the right way? Oh shit where are we?

As usual I hadn't taken enough notice of where Jack had taken me so once again I was lost somewhere in the middle of the very big council estate. I felt sick and foolish, which transferred to Poppy, who started walking even faster as if she could sense I had no idea where we were. I dread to think what she was thinking but I'd imagine it contained several swear words. She snorted as if expressing her distrust in me and I tried to slow her down without much success. Finally, round the next bend I realised where we were and breathed a big sigh of relief. Poppy felt me relax so she slowed down.

We were now on the main road that ran along the far edge of the estate. It was a very long, straight road with a wide grass verge and strangely the presence of so many cars had a calming effect on Poppy and she walked very nicely up the hill.

'Trot on!' I commanded, suddenly feeling brave. Poppy went into her extraordinarily fast trot and thundered up the road, round the bend and onto the road that led back to the yard.

'Yay! We did it, Poppy! Good girl.' I patted her neck and breathed a deep sigh of relief.

But we haven't cantered! I need to know I can do that on my own too. I'll just take her up the grass by the side of the road here, I thought to myself nonchalantly.

The grassy area by the dual carriageway, opposite the yard entrance, was wide enough and long enough to be a field really. It had several trees dotted about and it looked like a great place for our first solo canter. So instead of going straight across towards the yard gate, I asked Poppy to turn right instead. As if reading my mind, Poppy went into a canter.

'Aaaand whoa!' A few strides of canter were enough for me to know that I was capable of cantering alone.

'Whoaaa!' I repeated as Poppy shifted a gear and went faster.

'Oh my God!' I shrieked as she flew up the grass. Trees zipped past us and she upped the pace and exploded into a gallop.

'Nooooo!' I yelled.

Faster and faster she ran.

'Whoa! Whoa!' I pleaded.

The wind whipped my face, making my eyes stream. On my

left was the suddenly very busy dual carriageway. Ahead of us was the massive roundabout where the main road met an even busier A road. I felt sick and suddenly roasting hot. My heart was thumping in my throat. I clung onto the reins, crippled by the realisation that I had no idea how to stop her.

'We're going to die!' I screamed. The roundabout loomed before me with lorries thundering along the road towards it.

'Stooooop!' I shouted and suddenly she screeched to a halt. I lurched out of the saddle onto her neck, hung on for a moment and then fell sideways onto the grass with a loud thud.

I sobbed, mainly from the shock of the whole thing but also because I felt completely idiotic. Poppy looked down at me apologetically. I could almost hear her saying, 'I thought that's what you wanted me to do?'

After what felt an age, I dragged myself to my feet and with shaky hands I ran the stirrups up and took hold of the reins to lead her home. My arms were as heavy as lead and I felt like an absolute prat.

What possessed me to canter her up the grass near the yard? Of course she was going to go super-fast, she wanted to get back home! Why am I so stupid?

With jelly legs, I tottered back up the long driveway, into the barn and collapsed onto a chair.

'Oh hello, Grace,' cooed the sarcastic voice of Louise. 'I was just driving into the yard when I saw the most ridiculous sight I've ever seen. I saw a total fool on a large chestnut mare, galloping uncontrollably towards the roundabout. Can you imagine anyone being stupid enough to do that?' She laughed and walked off to take her horse into the school, leaving me feeling utterly wretched.

Poppy looked genuinely upset by the whole experience and stood quietly as I struggled to untack her with unwieldy fingers, swollen like sausages. I wanted to get out of there as quickly as possible before anyone else could see what a mess I was in. Luckily, all was still quiet as I hurried to put my things away. I dashed to my car and drove home feeling horrendous beyond measure.

I had never been more relieved to stumble into my kitchen, make a cup of chamomile tea and sit down at the table. My entire being was so shocked I couldn't think straight, which was a slight comfort. I wanted to call my mum but felt guilty that I'd been horse riding when I could have spent that time doing something nice with her. She did so much for me and never asked for anything in return. But then suddenly, something inspired me to check my work diary and to my horror I discovered I had mistakenly thought I had no one booked in when in fact I had Lady Alexa Heptonstall due to arrive in half an hour. I was like a whirlwind, tidying, cleaning and vacuuming the kitchen, stairways, landings and finally my therapy room. This was the route my clients had to take so it all had to be presentable. I tore my riding clothes off, hurled them on my bedroom floor, dragged my work clothes on and had a few seconds spare to splash some water on my face and tie my hair in a ponytail.

'I can almost hear you thinking,' Alexa tinkled in her cut-glass voice, halfway through the massage.

'What do you mean?' I asked.

'It's no use trying to pretend you're ok just because you're working. You can't fool me. So come on, spit it out! What's happened, old thing? I could tell by the way you waddled up the stairs that you've fallen off your horse,' she chuckled.

'Oh heck,' I sighed. 'It's not really very professional for me to talk about myself when it's your massage. You're not paying me to listen to my rubbish.'

'I don't mind in the least. It will make a very pleasant change to hear about someone else's disaster rather than my own,' she laughed.

'Ok, well if you're sure?'

'I insist. Now get on with it!'

I poured out the entire morning. How I hadn't taken any notice of the notice board when everybody else had. How I had no idea about worming a horse. And the grand finale – how I foolishly cantered up a dual carriageway with no control whatsoever.

'... and then she stopped suddenly and that's when I fell off. And to make matters worse, the yard bitch saw it all and made nasty comments about it,' I admitted, blushing with embarrassment.

Lady Alexa sat up and grinned. 'So now I expect you're beating yourself up and thinking how terrible a rider you are and you shouldn't have this type of horse? Am I right?'

'Yes.' I was impressed by her astute mind.

'Well you listen to me,' she folded her arms and looked very serious, 'I think you are a very brave woman.'

'Brave? I think I'm a prize idiot.'

'Not at all! Look where you began. You started out riding steady little cobs at a very safe little yard with a small group of middle-aged lovely women who just rode for fun. And here you are now with this stunning young sports horse at a much bigger yard full of competitive riders. Not only that but you have taken on a horse that's clearly had a bad start and you are helping her to improve.'

I nodded my head but still felt crap.

'We all make mistakes. Owning a horse is a never-ending life lesson. Believe me, you'll have plenty more bad experiences as you go forwards. But what you need to do is have more faith in yourself. You stayed on while she was moving and you managed to stop her just in time.'

'Yes, eventually when I shouted "Stop!" really loudly,' I sighed. 'It's not great horsemanship. It was just luck.'

'Well it worked. Maybe she understands the word stop? Experiment with it and see if it works in other situations,' suggested Alexa. 'And as for your yard bitch, there's one at every yard. They take great pleasure in undermining other people's confidence because they have very little going on in their own sad lives. Don't give her another thought.'

'I know you're right. I need to ignore her. I'm also really worried about moving to a field with no one to ride with except Jack. And ever since I bought Poppy I have to admit, I've begun to feel really – damn what's the word? Immature? That might not be the right description but you know, I just feel completely out of my depth with all the things I don't know. The responsibility of owning a horse. I feel the way I felt when I was a child. That's the word – I feel childish.'

'I think I understand what you're trying to say. All I can say is that I've begun to believe that each horse is sent to us so we can learn something important about ourselves. I wonder if there was something in your childhood that was unfinished perhaps? Something you didn't do but needed to?'

'That's very deep.'

'Yes it is. Horses take us into the depths of ourselves if we let them. Just get back on tomorrow and go for a little walk alone. Do it every day but keep it short, even if it's only five minutes and then build it up. I think you just did too much too soon that's all.' Alexa was full of wisdom and I felt very lucky to know her.

Later that evening my mind floated back to the conversation with Alexa. I pondered on the potential lesson that Poppy might be presenting me with but all I could feel was fear at the prospect of being somewhere with nobody to ride with most of the time. Fear of her erratic behaviour and fear of how much it was all costing. This was not how my childhood dream of owning a pony had looked in my mind for all those years. I was annoyed at myself for wallowing in self-pity, so I forced myself to get up and do some housework to distract myself.

Chapter 6

Winter was fast approaching and we had got nowhere with the new field due to Jack getting caught up in a very big joinery job that seemed to keep growing daily.

'The weather's too bad now for me to start building the shelter and I don't want to just chuck the horses onto a bare field,' said Jack as I led Poppy into the middle of the barn to tie her at the bar. 'It's a shame though. I love it there and really wanted to be on by now.'

'Well it's ok, at least we know we have it. I've told Valentina we're waiting until spring and she said that's fine. Fingers crossed they will have sorted out those ponies before then. I'd prefer them to be gone before we come on.'

'Yes, me too.' Jack nodded. 'It's really not our place to sort out a woman who won't pay them rent. I wouldn't put up with that, would you? I mean really, you'd just chuck her off.'

'I'd take the ponies to her house and put a padlock on the field gate so she couldn't bring them back,' I laughed.

'Hell yes,' agreed Jack. I prepared Poppy's grooming tools while Jack dashed off to work.

I had yet to venture out alone since my mishap because each time I tried there had always been someone there who wanted to ride with me. It was very nice but I realised that it wasn't helping me get over my fear of riding alone.

'Right, Miss Poppy.' I looked her in the eye. She looked back at me. 'Today we are going to walk across into the estate and then come back without any drama, ok?' Poppy breathed deeply as if unconcerned.

It felt extremely uncomfortable to mount on my own in the silence of the barn. It took a few minutes for me to pluck up the courage to walk up the steps to the mounting block. I took the reins in my left hand and put my right hand on the saddle.

God she can run so fast. What if she thinks that I am wanting her to gallop up the grass again when we cross over it? Nausea washed over me.

Just shut up and get on! Remember that she will relax if you relax!

Memories of my time in Wales flooded back and I took a deep breath and imagined myself feeling very calm. With some trepidation, I put my foot in the stirrup and mounted.

I am a very relaxed person, walking along a quiet, woodland path. I am feeling soooo chilled out.

Poppy responded and walked leisurely down the driveway to the gate that led to the road opposite the council estate.

'Good girl, Poppy. We'll go across the very wide stretch of grass, into the estate, up the first road and then we'll come back.' I breathed deeply.

As soon as her foot touched the first blade of grass my brain went on red alert. My body became rigid and a cold sweat began to form on my forehead. Ears pricked and ready for flight, Poppy responded to my anxiety by walking very fast with her head high. This fed back to my brain and made me breathe fast and shallow. My arms began to feel very heavy and nausea began to rise.

I've got to get off.

No! Don't be silly, you can do this.

No I can't! Why did I buy this horse? She's too much for me!

Remember what Julie said. Just think differently.

I found it impossible to control my spiralling fears and held tight on the reins, which made poor Poppy lift her head higher. She tried to speed up to get away from whatever I was terrified of but my hands pulled her back. It was like a battle against each other that neither of us could win. Her strides became short and choppy and as soon as we had made it over the grass to the other side, I leaped off.

'Bloody hell,' I sighed and took a few moments to steady myself. Poppy relaxed instantly and nosed at the ground so I ran her stirrups up and sat down on somebody's garden wall. I held my head in my hands and felt like a total failure.

'Eh up lass,' greeted a familiar voice. 'What's going on here then?' It was Jim, the settled traveller, who had rescued me the first time I had got lost in the sprawling council estate several months ago.

'Oh thank God it's you.' I almost cried with relief when I saw the old man. 'I'm such an idiot,' I wailed.

'Why?' asked Jim, his dark eyes widening behind his wire-rimmed glasses. 'What's happened, luv?'

'I don't feel capable of owning this sort of horse!' I blurted.

"Why ever not??' asked Jim, taking Poppy's reins and stroking her neck.

'I don't feel that I'm experienced enough to deal with all her needs and riding her on my own is terrifying. But I have to ride her on my own because we're moving soon and there won't always be someone to ride with like there is here.' I poured out the embarrassing story of my previous solo ride.

'Oh dear. Sounds like we need to have a good chat. Come on, we'll go to my house and I'll teach yer a bit about this type of horse.' Jim smiled and ran his hand through his thick curly black hair.

Relieved, I walked with Jim to his house while he led Poppy, and on the way, I explained more about how I had been feeling since I became her official owner. The rugs, the worming, the potential need for physio – all the things I hadn't known about that had made me feel like an absolute imbecile. Presently, we arrived at his house and he led Poppy into his large back garden where she immediately began to graze. Jim climbed up the steps of his traditional Romany caravan and invited me to follow.

'I love it in here, it's so colourful. I wish I could have something like this,' I sighed.

Everything had been restored to the glories of yesteryear with lots of burgundy, red and pink velvet soft furnishings and gold trimmings all over the place. In contrast, the roof was painted a vibrant yellow and green. We sat near a wood burning stove, next to a dark wooden dresser which had a beautifully embroidered linen cloth on the top. Jim brewed some tea and put out some biscuits on a fancy china plate adorned with blue, hand-painted roses.

'Last time I saw you, you were only loaning Poppy. Now you've obviously bought her so what's getting you so worked up?'

'I assumed that once I was her owner, I would feel different,' I said.

'What do you mean by that?' asked Jim kindly, sitting back into the plump luxurious cushions and folding his arms across his chest.

'I don't know. I suppose just more in control and confident,' I replied.

'Now listen to me, young lady. That's the daftest thing I ever heard in my life,' he grinned widely. 'It's not like in a fairy tale where they suddenly all live happily ever after you know. This horse has come to you for a reason and it's not just about riding neither. It's about a lifetime of learning. Ok, so you didn't know about rugs and this and that. But you do now don't you?'

'Yes,' I agreed, remembering Alexa's similar words.

'And riding on your own just takes time and patience. I wouldn't even ride her at first. Take the pressure off yourself and just walk with her if you're worried. I used to walk all my horses a few miles a day, every day for months until I could tell they felt confident being out on their own with me. And even after that when they were good riding horses, I always made sure I regularly took them for a walk. It's always important.'

'Really?' I asked with great surprise. 'You just walked them?' I suddenly remembered my lesson with Elise where we had walked Poppy in-hand and I wished I'd done more of it.

'Aye, I walked them because it was a great bonding experience,' Jim replied. 'Look at it from her point of view. She's a herd animal. That means she feels safer in a group of her own kind. Why should she feel happy going away from them on her own with just you? You need to show her she is ok on her own with you and that will only come with miles of walking, together.'

I pondered on his words for a few moments. 'What I don't understand is, I learned so much from this amazing horse woman, in Wales, about how to use my body language to help Poppy relax, but I just don't seem to be able to do it on my own,' I lamented.

Jim chuckled and shook his head. 'You need to practise these things a thousand times before it comes naturally. You're expecting a bit much of yourself too soon, lass. That Welsh lady has probably been working with horses every day for most of her life.'

'Yes, I suppose I'd not considered that.' It slowly dawned on me that as with everything in life, practice makes progress. I'd been expecting the magic I had learned in Wales with Julie to instantly transform me, yet I hadn't put enough time into actually doing it.

'Do you know what I'd do if I were you? I'd spend a few minutes riding in the school practising the body language stuff and then I'd take her for a short walk, in-hand. Do it regular and you'll soon be ready for when you move to yer new place.' Jim poured another cup of tea and we sat in silence for a while just looking out of the window at Poppy grazing.

'This type of horse is very sensitive, but they want to have a job,' said Jim eventually, breaking the silence. 'They usually get ruined by idiots who just want them to gallop all o'er the place and jump when they're too young and their bodies are still growing. She probably thought you wanted her to go hell fer leather up the grass because some daft bugger will have done that with her when she were about two, I reckon.'

'Really? Do you think that's what they did?' I was horrified at the thought of it.

'I'd bet my life on it. A lot of breeders want to produce a fast competition type of horse really quickly so they can mek as much money as possible. They get young kids to gallop an' jump 'em so they can put photos on Facebook showing how high the horse can jump. Like that's all that matters, bloody idiots. That's when good horses get ruined.'

'That's awful.' I shook my head.

'Yes it is. But your Poppy is still young enough to recover and become a good family horse. If she were a really nervy animal, she wouldn't be wandering around my garden eating everything like she is. Just watch her now. She's very happy on her own, isn't she? I think you're just worrying too much. I know your type – too many thoughts! Stop thinking and start doing. But do it slowly and don't expect an overnight miracle.'

'You're very wise,' I replied. 'I'm really glad I met you!'

Jim laughed his head off. 'I reckon you're the first person to ever say that.'

'Am I an idiot to have a horse like this when all I want to do is hack?' I remembered the nasty remarks Louise had made. 'Should I have got a cob instead?'

'I know what you mean,' Jim replied thoughtfully. 'It's a bit like trying to mek a sow's ear out of a purse when it's usually the other way round. But no, I actually don't think you're an idiot. Yes, she's been bred for competitions but she's got a more relaxed side to her than most sport horses. We can see that clear enough here. Just look at her. What do you see?'

'I see a very relaxed horse eating your garden.'

'Aye. Happy on her own. Most young horses of her type would definitely not be happy to wander round someone's garden on their own.'

'Really?'

'Yes, really. They'd be pacing up and down calling out.'

'Right.' I nodded. 'I feel so much better for seeing you.' I smiled.

'I'm very glad to hear it, young lady. Now let's walk her home together and see how she is on these roads in hand.'

Jim took an old lead rope out of a drawer and we went in to the garden to get Poppy. 'It's easier to lead them with a rope, rather than reins, so she can lower her head and relax more,' he explained, attaching the rope to her bridle. 'But always use your bridle in case you need more control. Now you walk by her right shoulder and relax your own shoulders, they're up by yer ears!'

Eventually, we were ready to go and we walked around the roads, letting Poppy have a good look at different cars, driveways, bikes and lots of people walking past. She was very interested in everything and she was clearly feeling very safe. I felt relaxed because I had the calming presence of Jim and the walk back to the yard was very enjoyable.

'Now, you're lucky because whoever started her got her well used to traffic. She's not bothered at all so she must have been on a lot of busy roads. I think you'll be fine walking her round the estate and you know where I live if you get worried.' Jim smiled.

'Thank you. You are the horse angel.' I grinned.

'Now I've never been called an angel before,' he laughed and shook his head. 'Give her a few carrots and give yourself a pat on the back. And let me know how it's going. Pop in next week or so.'

'Thank you, I will.' I smiled widely and led a very relaxed Poppy up the drive. Just in time to pass Louise who was leaving the yard. She stopped her car and wound her window down.

'Did you fall off again?' she smirked.

'No, we are bonding,' I replied, feeling strangely calm.

'Bonding? That's the sort of ridiculous thing Alex would say. She's a horse. She needs to just do what she's told.' She wound her window up and drove away.

'Well,' I laughed out loud. 'I bet you're glad you're not her horse. Silly cow,' I said to Poppy, who was completely oblivious.

I took Poppy into her stable to untack and give her a good

brush all over. I felt elated to have been taught such wise words from a seasoned horseman. The responsibility of horse ownership began to feel a lot more doable thanks to Jim and I vowed to make an effort to remember it was lifelong learning and not to expect everything to suddenly be perfect.

And Louise can sod off too ...

Chapter 7

December arrived in its usual whirlwind kind of a way. Every day was packed with mum stuff, dog stuff, horse stuff and work. I was making great progress walking out with Poppy on my own and Jim had been a constant source of help. It felt like the fastest month of the year and I was too busy to notice it passing by until suddenly it was Boxing Day.

Normally, Boxing Day was all about making cups of tea and sandwiches for various relatives and it was usually a very exhausting day, but miraculously the universe had allowed me an escape this year. I had before me the rare opportunity to go for a ride. I was up, dressed and out of the door before anyone could change their mind and I leaped into the car with glee. It had snowed overnight, which added to the excitement of the moment. Isn't it amazing how a blanket of snow can transform mundane suburbia into a magical wonderland? The roads were quiet as I drove to the yard, marvelling at the beauty of the snow-covered trees that lined the way. It was like venturing out into Narnia.

Jack and Sally had suggested a fun ride to the village pub for the three of us and I was really looking forward to it.

'Oh for goodness' sake, Veronica! You can't ride in that dress, it's not very practical now is it?' came the thunderous tones of Morag as I stepped out of my car.

Morag was in the stable barn yet I could hear her as clear as day from the carpark, which was at least thirty yards away. I looked over with amusement, wondering what sight would befall me.

'Oh my God,' said Jack as she stormed out and strode over.

'We're all in for it now.'

Before I had time to ask her what she meant, Morag marched outside, climbed onto a decrepit trailer, cleared her throat and bellowed (without any need for a megaphone), 'Ok everyone! Gather round!'

Nobody dared to argue. Several people walked out of their stables and we all waited, like rabbits in headlights, wondering what on earth this announcement was going to be.

'As it's Boxing Day I thought we could all relive our pony club days and enjoy a treasure hunt. So, I have arranged for a trail to be laid and prizes are hidden along the way to make it even more jolly. Come along, everyone, let's get ready!'

Everyone stood, dumbstruck and jaws dropped open. I looked at Sally, expecting her to be the brave one and explain that we were going to the pub. But even Sally just gave a wilted smile and said, 'Great, thanks Morag. That will be fun.' So our fates were sealed.

Just at that moment, the slamming of a door startled us all back to life and we looked around to see Louise had arrived.

'I told you to park it facing the other way! How am I going to load my horse? You can see the ramp opens on the left. Honestly, why are you so stupid? Turn it around!' Louise, red-faced and furious, marched towards us, leaving her poor benighted husband to manoeuvre her vehicle.

'Hello everybody,' she greeted us curtly. 'What's going on? Why is everybody standing outside?'

Morag jumped off the trailer.

'Good morning, Louise,' said Morag very enthusiastically. 'I have arranged a Boxing Day treasure hunt. It's going to be tremendous fun for everyone!'

'Oh really? Well I won't be joining you for that childish nonsense. I'm going on a real Boxing Day hunt followed by a cocktail party at the manor house.' And with that she walked off to feed and groom her unfortunate horse, leaving Morag looking slightly stunned.

'It's a Christmas miracle! Thank the gods and goddesses she's not coming,' laughed Alex. 'I love treasure hunts. Thanks for sorting it, Morag!'

'You would love treasure hunts,' muttered Jack as she wandered off to her van to get her saddle.

'I think this is going to be fun,' chuckled Sally. 'I haven't done anything like this since I was ten.'

I was beginning to feel quite enthusiastic about it too. I had very fond memories of doing a Boxing Day treasure hunt at the riding school when I was young, which had been excellent.

'Morning ladies.' Danny had just arrived, looking gorgeous as ever. 'What's going on?'

'Oh Danny, I'm glad you're here. You can help make sure everyone has got enough high viz to be safe for the treasure hunt. We certainly don't want any accidents now do we?' and she marched a bemused looking Danny off to her stable.

'Crikey Alex! What's happened to your horse? She looks like a Christmas tree.' I couldn't believe my eyes as Alex led Giant Jenny out of her stable. She was covered in tinsel and wearing a headband with antlers on. 'I don't think you'll be needing to wear any high viz with all that lot.'

'Indeed not, for I am wearing my elf costume,' Alex replied, unzipping her coat to reveal that she really was dressed as an elf.

'God help us all,' sighed Jack, shaking her head.

Poppy took an instant dislike to the glittery tinsel, snorting and rolling her eyes as if it were a monster. She refused to come out of her stable and reversed right up to the back wall and planted her feet.

'Oh nightmare,' I muttered as my heart dropped. We had been doing so well recently, I wasn't prepared for a setback.

'Come on, Poppy, let's go,' I said, pulling slightly on her lead rope and trying to sound cheery.

She pulled back, her head high in the air and her eyes white with fear. She was glued to the ground. 'Walk on!' I said firmly, trying to keep myself calm. Poppy yanked her head to the side and refused to move. I realised I couldn't force her to move, she weighed half a ton.

What the hell am I going to do? I wish Jim were here! He'd know exactly what to do. I felt panic rising as I realised I might not be able to ride after all. I began to feel very hot and embarrassed as I had no idea how to deal with this situation. None of the other horses seemed remotely bothered by Jenny's decorations so I didn't understand why Poppy was behaving like this.

'Come on, Poppy, it's ok,' I pleaded.

I could feel my heart beating and my breathing became shallow.

If you're worried, she'll be worried, interjected the wise part of my brain. Memories of Julie, from Wales, pinged into my head.

What would she do in this situation? She wouldn't be pulling on a lead rope that's for sure. What would she do, though? She would do the opposite of pull. She would probably sit down and have a cup of tea.

I walked out of the stable, took a deep breath and relaxed my body as if to say, 'Actually, I'm not worried about this and I don't care if you stay in your stable all day.' I sat on an upturned bucket and pretended to file my nails. Then I had the bright idea of going over to Jenny and touching her decorations. I wrapped some of the tinsel around my neck like a scarf and glanced over to Poppy. She snorted and looked absolutely horrified as if I had completely lost my mind and I laughed at her expression. My laughter must have helped her to realise it was ok because she suddenly relaxed her posture and took a step forward.

'Good girl,' I said with great relief and I played around with the tinsel just far enough away for Poppy to feel safe yet be able to see clearly that it was ok.

'Here, Grace, take her this carrot with the tinsel,' said Alex passing me a carrot.

Poppy could never resist a carrot, even if it was wrapped in scary tinsel. She snuffled around in the tinsel and found the carrot. While she ate it, I dangled the tinsel over my head and then I draped it around her neck. She lifted her head high for a few moments but then relaxed as she realised that it wasn't going to hurt her. She almost looked a bit sad when I took it off her.

'You can keep it,' laughed Alex. 'I think she wants to wear it!'

I tied the green garland of tinsel around her neck and Poppy looked very smug. It certainly was a lovely contrast to her ginger fur. I was so enormously relieved about it I did a little dance as I got my grooming kit out.

'Well done, Poppy. You are so brave,' I said, kissing her cheek. Poppy looked like she almost smiled.

'How funny that you were worried about tinsel yet you don't give a stuff about double-decker buses driving past us,' I mused as I led her out of her stable and tied her at the bar in the centre of the barn.

'Have you put the ramp down?' spat Louise to her husband in the most caustic voice she could muster. I felt very sorry for him as he muttered something and scuttled off to the horsebox like a scolded hen. It was bad enough sharing a livery yard with Louise. I certainly would not want to be sharing a life with her too.

Today Louise was very smartly dressed in a black hunting jacket, white breeches and boots that were so shiny it hurt my eyes to look at them. No doubt her poor husband had the job of cleaning those. I imagined she stood over him with an electric cattle prod at the ready in case he wasn't polishing them to her standard.

'Hark the herald angels sing,' sang Veronica in her terrible opera style as she rode out of the barn, side-saddle. She was wearing a long, flowing, dark-green velvet Edwardian gown that she must have got from a fancy-dress shop. It looked slightly odd teamed with wellies and a jockey skull cap with a lilac silk.

'That woman needs to be sectioned,' sniffed Louise as she marched her horse out towards her horsebox.

'Thank God she isn't coming with us,' I said to Alex, who agreed heartily.

'Is everybody ready?' bellowed Morag.

Everyone was more or less ready to be inspected by Morag, the self-appointed health and safety-officer. Morag was wearing a brand-new, fluorescent yellow jacket with a very interesting message on the back which I initially read as 'Police'.

What the hell? I thought to myself and had a second look.

It actually said, 'Polite! Please pass wide and slow!' and all around the bottom edge were blue and white checks. Coupled with her blue and white checked hat band she looked exactly like a mounted police officer. I had to bite my hand to stop guffawing out loud with hysterical laughter. Just as we were all mounting up, June came rolling in in her wheelchair.

'Merry Boxing Day!' she called out cheerily. 'Where are you all going?'

'Merry Boxing Day, June,' I replied. 'Morag has arranged a treasure hunt.'

June looked wistfully at all of us going out on the treasure hunt. 'Oh I wish I could come,' she said sadly. 'It would be a dream come true.'

'I don't think you should go out riding in the snow,' said her husband, David, looking very worried.

'I know, but I really do want to go,' sighed June.

'I don't think it's a good idea with your back,' replied David firmly.

'But it's not too bad today actually.' June stood up and wiggled her hips, her eyes alight with hope. 'And Beatrix has been behaving well with the Western trainer, she hasn't reared for weeks. The doctor says I'm doing much better too.'

'Yes and we want to keep it that way, don't we dearest?' her poor husband almost pleaded.

'Oh David you only live once. Do you know what? Bugger it, I'm riding!'

David looked very flustered and unhappy but he knew it would be pointless arguing with June once she'd made her mind up. All he could do was pray she would be ok.

'Morag, you all go on ahead and me, Grace, Sally and Alex will help June,' said Jack.

'Ok. Here is the list of clues.' Morag handed Jack the list.

'To horse, everyone! To horse!' and everyone else mounted and clattered off.

Getting Beatrix and June ready to go didn't take too long between all of us and presently we were all mounted and riding out into the snow. The sky was blue and the sun was shining and I suddenly felt the way I had when I was a child at the riding school doing the Boxing Day treasure hunt.

'Right, the first clue is absolutely meaningless,' said Jack, already exasperated by the whole thing.

'Here, pass it over,' I said as Jack handed me the list. 'I love things like this. Oh God, what?'

'Exactly,' grumbled Jack.

'What does it say?' asked Alex.

'It says *Follow your nose to the old oak tree but don't be put off by the smell.* I have no idea what that means,' I laughed.

Sally and Alex laughed their heads off because it sounded so mad.

'Ooh that's easy,' said June.

'Easy?' I asked.

'It's the pig farm isn't it? You know the one I mean surely?'

'Oh yes!' we all said together.

'And there's a right big old oak tree in their field.'

'Oh heck do we have to go in a field with a load of pigs?' I was horrified. 'Poppy will explode!'

'Surely not,' said Jack. 'Let's go over there and have a look and if the pigs are out we'll go to the pub instead.' We all agreed except Alex, who really wanted to do the whole ride, and off we went to the pig farm, which was not too far away.

Riding through the village was a treat for the eyes. It was like being in a real live Christmas card. All the cottages were covered in fairy lights and they all had beautifully decorated Christmas trees in their windows. Lots of kids in bobble hats and mittens waved at Alex thanks to her crazy elf costume and decorated horse.

'You know, Christmas was originally a pagan festival,' said Alex, who loved all things magical. 'It wasn't anything like what people do these days.'

'Here we go,' sighed Jack under her breath. 'Do tell me more, Alex. What was it really about then?'

'It was about lighting up the dark winter and making merry,' replied Alex.

'Right,' said Jack. 'So a bit like what everybody is actually doing now then?'

'Yes, I suppose so,' laughed Alex.

'Seriously, God give me strength,' muttered Jack. It was always entertaining to listen to Alex and Jack.

'There's the tree!' shouted June, gleefully.

Luckily the giant oak tree wasn't far from the wall and the pigs weren't in the field. It still absolutely stank of pigs though, due to all their little sheds dotted about the field. Poppy snorted. She didn't relish the scent and I couldn't blame her.

'Ok, who's going to be mad enough to have a look in the field?' asked Jack.

'Meee!' shouted Alex as she leaped down from her horse, bells jingling on her outfit. She tripped over her own feet and bashed her head on the wall.

'Oh for the love of God,' sighed Jack.

'I'm alright,' Alex laughed and pulled herself up. Jenny, her horse simply stood still as if nothing had happened.

'So do you need to go to the oak tree?' I asked. 'Is the treasure in the tree?'

Alex climbed over the wall and headed for the tree.

'There's a bag!' she shouted. 'Oh hahaaa! It's full of chocolate coins!'

'Brilliant!' shouted Sally. 'Don't let Malcy see them, though. He'll eat them! He loves chocolate.'

'Don't we all?' I laughed at the thought of Malcy eating chocolate.

Alex almost had to hurl herself back over the wall. She wasn't the most athletic of people but she was so enthusiastic.

'Chocolate for everyone but not for you, Malcy.' She handed us all a chocolate coin.

'What's the next clue?' asked June.

'Oh good God,' said Jack. 'It says *Head for the woods next. Who let the dogs out? Careful not to get told off!* What the hell does that mean?'

'That's so mad,' I laughed my head off.

'Dog Kennel Lane! The racehorse training place!' shrieked Alex with great excitement. 'Come on!'

'But that's miles away from here,' grumbled Jack. 'Why would that be the next place?'

'I don't know but what else can it be? We always get told off when we try to sneak a canter down their gallops track,' replied Alex.

'That's true,' agreed Jack. 'Ok everyone, let's go. June how are you feeling?'

In all the excitement I had completely forgotten that June was a disabled rider. Luckily she was fine, and so far there had been no hijinks with her horse, Beatrix. We set off for the racing stables and as we entered the woods, large snowflakes began to fall softly from the sky.

'Have a holly jolly Christmas!' I sang.

'It's the best time of the year!' joined in Sally.

It was such excellent fun riding in the snow looking for mad clues and singing that we all let go of our inhibitions and laughed like we were kids again. Memories of my riding school days flooded my mind as I revelled in the fact my childhood dream had finally come true. Here I was riding along on a horse that was mine. I never thought that would ever happen.

'Aaarghhhh!' yelled June as Beatrix reared up.

Shocked, I turned round to see a black horse thunder past with a ghostly rider wearing dark billowing clothes. This was too much for Poppy, who leaped sideways, snorted loudly and broke into a very fast canter.

'Whoa!' I called out as she began to speed up. 'Steady now! Whoaa!'

I was terrified we would crash as trees flashed past. I clung onto the reins and sat deep into the saddle. The air filled with expletives as, behind me, all the horses freaked out and began running. I feared the most for June and that thought helped me to feel calm, in control and slow Poppy down.

'Stoooooop! Poppy, for God's sake you'll kill June!' I shouted .

Poppy slowed immediately and stopped. Something inside me was ready for this so instead of flying out of the saddle like I had done previously, I leaned back, and although I lurched forwards and landed on her neck I managed to stay on. I looked around and everyone else screeched to a halt, almost crashing into us.

'Jesus Christ,' gasped Alex, fanning herself. 'I don't think Jenny's ever moved that fast in her life!'

'I don't think Malcy's ever moved that fast either,' laughed Sally. 'He'll need a rest now.'

Poor Malcy was breathing very deeply and looked rather annoyed. Running fast was not his favourite pass time.

'I stayed on!' shouted June, laughing with relief. 'I stayed ON!'

'Thank God for that. You did really well.' I was enormously relieved. I was terrified that June would fall off and be unable to walk ever again. 'Who the hell was that galloping past us? That's so bloody rude!' I was furious.

'I'll give you three guesses.' Jack, who had seen who it was, grimaced. 'But you have to sing her name in an opera style.'

'No way! Was it Veronica?'

'Yep. Bloody lunatic she is. Now we are lost thanks to her and the snow is falling heavier.'

I looked around and realised Jack was right. I had no idea where we were and neither did anyone else.

'We'll just have to keep riding forwards in a straight line and hope that we eventually get to a road,' said sensible Sally.

It was getting difficult to see as big, fat snowflakes kept hitting me in my eyes. Sadly, the fun had melted away and anxiety welled up in its place. Everyone was grumbling and cursing Veronica.

'What was the snowman doing in the vegetable patch?' asked Alex.

'Pardon?' I thought I'd misheard her.

'I said, what was the snowman doing in the vegetable patch?' she repeated.

'I have no bloody idea, Alex,' replied Jack.

'Picking his nose!' Alex laughed her head off, which made us all laugh and the mood was lifted.

'That's such a shit joke,' I chuckled.

'I know,' she laughed.

'The hunt!' shouted Jack.

'The what?' I asked.

'The hunt! Listen!' in the distance I heard the traditional huntsman's horn.

'Oh no. That's all we need.' My heart began thumping. I had visions of Poppy going mad and racing after the hunt.

'We need to go steady and carefully,' said Sally. 'We don't want to get mixed up in all of that.'

With ears pricked up, we all rode as quietly as we could, listening out for where the hunt might be. After a while, the woods thinned out and eventually ended and we found ourselves in some scrubland. Ahead of us, a bit lower down in a massive field, were the members of the hunt streaming away into the distance. We breathed a collective sigh of relief.

'Look! There's Louise!' shouted Alex.

'Where?' I asked. I couldn't have picked out anyone.

'Oh yes,' laughed Sally. 'She's at the back.'

Sure enough, lolloping along at the back was Louise. Her horse was looking pretty tired and was ignoring Louise's kicks to get her to hurry up.

'That poor horse. She must have some bad karma to have ended up belonging to Louise,' sighed Alex.

'Oh my God!' we all chorused.

From apparently nowhere, Veronica had appeared. Her crazy Edwardian dress blowing up in the air as her horse flew across the field to join the hunt. Louise's horse took one look at the dress and let out an almighty squeal. She leaped sideways, spun round and bolted for all she was worth – in our direction.

'Oh my God!' we all chorused again.

'Hold on to your horses!' shouted Jack and we all grabbed hold of their reins. This was, luckily, completely unnecessary as our horses didn't actually react at all. They must have been frozen with shock. Either that or they were enjoying the entertainment.

'I hope she's going to stop,' I panicked.

'She's going to crash into us if she doesn't!' replied June.

Louise's horse pulled up just in time and Louise sailed beautifully over her head, somersaulting in the air and landing with a resounding thud onto her bottom.

'Owwww!' she yelled in agony.

Kind-hearted Jack leaped off her horse and pulled Louise to her feet.

'Can you walk?' she asked.

'Not really. Ow bloody hell, my bum is killing me,' Louise began to cry.

Even though she was a total bitch, we couldn't help feeling sorry for her, which just goes to show that the heart is stronger than the mind in situations like this. However, I do have to admit to feeling slightly amused at the sight of Louise looking very dishevelled with a wet bottom. She looked like she had pissed herself.

'Bloody Veronica. I could kill her,' sniffed Louise. 'She needs to be locked up! I'm going to miss the post-hunt party now.' Louise began to sob hysterically as if the party was the most important thing in the world.

'That's the least of your worries.' I nodded. 'You landed really hard on your bottom. If you've broken your coccyx you won't be able to sit down for months.'

'Oh no,' cried Louise, her usually perfect face smeared with tears and snot.

'Here,' said Sally, passing her a tissue. 'Let's try and get home.'

'Where is the nearest road?' asked June.

Luckily it wasn't that far, but it wasn't much of a road. It was merely a quiet country lane and none of us had any phone signal. Louise was finding it extremely difficult to walk and it wasn't that easy for me and Sally as we both had horses to lead.

'I can't go on,' cried Louise, dramatically. 'I'm in agony!'

'Hmm,' said June, who knew all about pain. 'You haven't had a baby yet have you, love? Believe me, a broken arse bone is nothing compared to childbirth.'

We all nodded in agreement. But it was irrelevant for Louise, who didn't have the faintest idea what June was talking about. All she knew was her bottom was excruciatingly painful and home was a long way off.

'You have to keep going,' insisted Jack, almost dragging her along. 'There's no other option. We'll get some signal soon and we can phone for help.'

'What's that over there?' I asked, suddenly noticing a flash of fluorescent yellow in the distance.

'It's Morag!' cried Sally excitedly. 'MOOOORRRAAAAAG!'

Poppy jumped out of her skin.

'Christ! You've deafened me! How on earth can you shout that loud?' My ears were ringing.

'I've got a teenage daughter so I need to be loud,' laughed Sally.

Miraculously, Morag heard Sally's shout and she and Danny came galloping over to us.

'Goodness me! What's happened to you?' blurted Morag when she saw Louise.

'Long story, but the short version is her horse got spooked by Veronica and her idiotic dress,' explained Alex.

'Oh dear oh dear. She needs an ambulance. Have you got signal? I haven't got any signal.' The flustered Morag started shaking her phone in the vain hope that would help.

'I don't think shaking your phone is going to make it work, Morag. But here comes a taxi,' said Danny.

Seeing the taxi approaching, as if from nowhere, was like a wonderful mirage.

'Halt!' shouted Morag, manoeuvring her horse into the middle of the road, holding her hand up to stop the taxi.

It was a very brave move considering the snowy circumstances. The taxi skidded to a halt, narrowly missing the lot of us.

'For God's sake, Morag,' blustered Jack as Buddy leaped sideways.

'Can I help you, officer?' asked the taxi driver, winding down his window.

'Officer? We need your assistance immediately!' instructed Morag. 'This lady is injured and needs to go to hospital as soon as possible!'

'But we are on our way to a party,' replied the passenger winding his window down. He was a very posh-looking middle-aged man wearing a very luxurious suede coat.

'I don't care if you are on your way to the moon! We are commandeering this taxi. This lady needs to go to hospital immediately!'

The man took one look at Morag and changed his tune.

'Oh! I'm terribly sorry. I didn't notice your uniform. Of course we must take her to hospital at once,' stuttered the man, red-faced.

Louise couldn't sit down so she had to lie across the back seat. Off they went to hospital while we all set off homeward.

'What did that man mean? My uniform?' asked Morag as the taxi drove away. 'And why did the taxi driver call me officer?'

We all looked open mouthed at Morag.

'Are you seriously asking that?' I laughed. 'You look like a mounted policewoman!'

Morag looked down at her jacket and saw the blue checks, quite possibly for the first time. It slowly dawned on her what she must look like.

'Oh! That's lucky isn't it?'

'How could you have not noticed?' Jack shook her head in disbelief.

The ride home was, thankfully, without any more incidents. David was almost in tears with relief when he saw June in one piece and none the worse for the adventure.

'All is well, David luv.' June grinned triumphantly. 'Madam reared up and she had a bit of a run but I managed absolutely fine. So I've decided to keep her and get some more lessons with the rodeo man.' David shook his head in resignation, but we could tell he was really very impressed with June's determination and courage.

The horses were rubbed down and were very happy to get back into their stables with feed buckets and haynets. I can only imagine what their take on the day was.

It had been the sort of experience the younger me would have relished. A ride brimming with the adventures of youth that rarely happen as an adult. I drove home grinning with a sense of achievement. I had managed to stop Poppy without falling off and the main thing was she clearly responded to the word *stop* rather than *whoa*, so I had that in my toolbox for any future shenanigans. I took a deep and happy breath as I realised I felt ready for the move to our own place.

Chapter 8

Jack fumbled in her pocket and pulled out a rather crumpled piece of paper and offered it to me. 'Right, have a look at this lot. We need all of this to build the shelter.'

'I don't actually know what any of this means,' I said, looking at the list.

'Don't worry, all you need to do is give me some cash and then I'll buy it and build it.' Jack grinned.

Spring had arrived with its promise of wonderful days to come and we felt the time was right to build the shelter. The field was waking up from its winter slumber. New green shoots of grass were coming through and all the hedges were coming into bud again. A flock of swallows were zipping around performing breath-taking aerobatics and yellow wagtails were bobbing around looking for worms. It was a glorious sight to behold. Unfortunately, the only blot on the landscape was that the three ponies were still there.

'What the hell are we going to do about them?' I wondered.

'God knows,' replied Jack, shaking her head. 'Let's just get on with the shelter and see what happens when we move on.'

The ponies looked very happy to see us and they were quite sweet really. There was a light bay of about 15hh, a grey of 14hh and a very young skewbald that looked to be about 12.2hh. They were very scruffy and clearly hadn't been groomed for months, as their manes were very knotty.

'Poor things,' I said as I gave one of them a pat.

'Right let's get on,' said Jack as she began measuring up the space for the shelter and marking out vital points. The sound of hooves approaching made the ponies prick their ears up and trot to the gate. I went with them to see who was coming.

A very glossy black horse, ridden by a middle-aged woman, hove into sight round the bend of the lane and when she reached our gate she stopped.

'Hello,' she greeted in a very friendly way. 'Are you friends of Anna?'

Jack had wandered over by this point. 'No we aren't!' she almost shouted. 'Do you know her?'

'Unfortunately, yes.' The lady pulled an irritated sort of a face.

'That doesn't sound good,' I replied. 'Why unfortunately?'

'She owes me quite a lot of money,' said the woman, twiddling her long, black plaits. Her dark eyes squinted in the sun.

'Oh, that's not good.' I shook my head. 'From the sounds of things, I don't think you'll be getting it anytime soon.'

'No, I probably won't. I used to have my horse on here with her and I ended up paying all the rent because she kept conveniently forgetting. And she kept promising to sort out the ragwort problem but never did. Anyway, I got fed up in the end so sadly I'm now at the farm opposite the pub.'

'That's really out of order,' said Jack. 'I refuse to let her get away with this any longer.'

'Well good luck with that.' The lady raised her eyebrows. 'She's a compulsive liar, so be ready for her coming up with every excuse under the sun as to why she can't pay. She'll tell you she has no money but don't fall for it. She's loaded. And she's got horses all over the place and she doesn't pay any rent anywhere!'

'What do you mean?' I asked, wide-eyed with surprise.

'She's got over twenty-five ponies and five fields that she

rents and never pays a penny because she plays the poverty card. She pretends she's a single mum and that her kids are ill so the landlords feel sorry for her. She hasn't even got any kids! She lives in a posh house in Bramhope and you should see her horse box, it's massive and almost new.'

'What an absolute cow! Well she's messing with the wrong people now.' Jack folded her arms and scowled.

'Good,' said the woman. 'It's about time someone stood up to her.' A tractor came round the corner so she said goodbye and trotted off.

'I'm not putting up with that,' said Jack angrily. 'Twenty-five ponies? That's insane. We need to let her know that we are absolutely not going to be taken for fools.'

'Yes,' I agreed. 'But how are we going to do that?'

'We're going to tell her she has to leave immediately,' said Jack. 'Let's send her a message now. Tell her we're moving our horses on in two weeks and she needs to be gone by then because we aren't putting up with her not paying rent. And say it really straight so she can see we mean business.'

I typed the message and pressed send, feeling a bit apprehensive. The reply came back immediately, 'I will move my ponies at the weekend.'

'Wow! Well that was easy enough,' I said.

'Great,' said Jack and she breathed a sigh of relief.

'What did that woman mean about "the ragwort problem"?' I wondered.

'I don't know,' shrugged Jack. 'I haven't noticed any, have you?'

'No.' I scanned the field and saw nothing.

'Right let's get on with this field shelter now. We'll worry about ragwort if it starts popping up.'

The weekend came and went.

'Those bloody ponies are still here,' grumbled Jack as we opened the gate on Monday morning to resume work on the shelter. 'She's taking the piss.'

'I'll call her,' I said, opening my phone and searching for her number. Anna didn't answer the phone but instead sent me a message.

'She says "my daughter broke her arm on Saturday and she needs an operation today to put pins in". What the hell?' I read out. Jack was too stunned to reply.

'I know that you don't have any children,' I said out loud as I typed my reply. 'So please come and remove your ponies. They must be out of here by next weekend as that is when we are moving our horses on.'

After a while of not getting a reply, Jack lost her temper and marched off to continue building the shelter. The ponies kept getting in her way, which wound her up even more. I shooed them off and went for a walk round the field to check where the water supply was as we hadn't thought of that until now. There was a water trough but no tap anywhere so I wandered over towards the house to see if there was an outside tap.

'Hallo!' called Valentina, making me jump. I looked around to find her on the patio. She was wearing a peach-coloured leotard with silver Lycra leggings and was balanced on a unicycle with a book on her head and arms outstretched. 'This is so amazing for core strength. Would you like to have a go?' She jumped off and the book landed in a water bowl that must have been the dog's.

'Er, no thanks. I was just wondering if there's a water supply for the field?' I asked.

'Oh yes! Come with me, I'll show you where it is,' and she walked with me to show me where it was, hiding on an old gate post under a thick clump of brambles. 'Oh there is your friend. She's very capable isn't she, building all that herself?' Valentina waved at Jack, who came over to say hello.

Jack looked very bemused at Valentina's outfit but managed to suppress the urge to laugh out loud. I could see she was about to go into convulsions so I hastily brought up the subject of Anna, knowing this would soon stop her from laughing.

'I'm not putting up with someone who won't pay their part of the rent,' fumed Jack. 'She needs to go, so we've given her until next weekend. Maybe you could also send her a message telling her she needs to be off by then?'

'Yes I will definitely do that. But if she won't go then I do not see what we can do.' Valentina shrugged her shoulders in a resigned sort of a way and went back to her unicycle.

'Why are they letting her get away with it?' asked Jack with annoyance when we were out of earshot. 'And what the hell was she wearing?' She burst out laughing.

'Valentina is a massive health fanatic.' I grinned. 'She's always doing really extreme things in the name of fitness.' I laughed as I recalled some of the crazy things she'd told me she had done. It was quite a treat to have finally seen her in action rather than just hearing about it though.

'What are we going to do if Anna doesn't move these ponies by the weekend? We can't let this go on, even if they aren't prepared to do anything,' said Jack.

'I have no idea,' I replied. 'Let's see what happens at the time and take it from there.'

The last week at Bob's livery yard was tinged with sadness. I had grown to love everyone (except Louise) and I was going to miss them. Although I felt more capable of riding out alone, I knew it wouldn't be the same without all the support I had there. I took Poppy over to see Jim for one last time.

'Well, I'm not going anywhere so you can always come and visit if you ever need to ask me anything.' He smiled brightly. 'I can see you've made great progress with Pop so you're ready to move on.' He patted Poppy's shoulder.

'I have, but I'm still a bit nervous about it all,' I replied.

'Have you ever heard that saying, "When the student is ready, the teacher will arrive"? It's always true. You met me here didn't you? Just trust that everything will work out for the best, because it will.'

I rode back to the yard pondering Jim's wise words. It was incredible how I had met him when I really needed someone who knew about horses. And I had met Elise when I needed a riding instructor and the wild women in Wales had manifested in a similar way. The more I thought about it the more peaceful I became and decided to trust fate. After dismounting and untacking I packed up all of Poppy's things. Isn't it amazing how much stuff you can accumulate without noticing it happening? I realised it was going to take more than one trip to drive everything over to the new field.

When I arrived with the first load, Jack was up a ladder putting the roof tiles on top of the shelter.

'It's too fucking high! Make it shorter!' came the sudden yell of the landlord, followed by a high-pitched squeak that sounded like feedback. We looked around but couldn't see him. Then came another piercing squeak followed by a loud crunchy, crackling noise. 'I can bloody see it from my bedroom window and I don't want to see that bastard eyesore! And keep the sodding noise down, I'm trying to work!' He was leaning out of a window at the top of his house shouting through a megaphone. We were stunned. It made another really loud crackling noise. 'Bloody hell. This fecking thing's broken now.' He disappeared back into the room.

'Oh my God, you've got to be joking,' spluttered Jack. 'How can I make it shorter now?' I was too dumbstruck to reply.

'Ey up! You've done a grand job, our lass,' Jack's dad walked through the field gate to marvel at the amazing structure his daughter had created. Jack climbed down her ladder and burst into tears.

'Eh luv! What's up?' asked her dad, as shocked as I was. I'd never seen Jack cry and clearly neither had her dad.

'The landlord has just told me to make it shorter! How the hell am I going to do that now?'

'What a bugger,' said her dad shaking his head. 'Don't you worry. I'll sort it.' He walked off to make a phone call while I gave Jack a tissue. She wasn't the hugging type. Ten minutes later, a big navy-blue Transit van pulled into the carpark and two of the most extraordinarily good-looking blokes leaped out. I was transfixed by their mocha skin and flashing green eyes and both of them were wearing tight t-shirts which showed off their perfectly muscular chests.

Jack smirked and prodded me. 'Come back to earth, Grace, these are my brothers.'

'Oh wow,' I stuttered.

'Seriously, Grace?' Jack shook her head. 'They're not wow, they're a couple of twats.'

'We are wow,' laughed the bigger of the two as I blushed.

'Now then, come on, lads, no time for flirting, we've got work to do,' chided the dad as he winked at me. 'I expect you're wondering how a man like me could produce such handsome kids eh?'

I didn't like to say but that was exactly what I was thinking.

'I often wonder what a beautiful, Jamaican woman saw in an ugly white, Yorkshire man like you, Dad,' chuckled Jack.

'It was my charm,' he laughed. 'Come on, lads, let's get to work.'

An assortment of tools and sets of ladders were hurled out of the back of the van. 'Luckily, we were on a job nearby,' said the slightly smaller brother.

I often wondered where workmen suddenly disappeared to in the middle of jobs and now I knew. It was like watching a miracle unfold as they worked out what to do and got on with sorting it out. Planks of wood were ripped off the sides and the top of the structure until eventually the upright beams were exposed, which were then shortened. The roof was then replaced and like magic, we had a fully functioning field shelter with lighting and store rooms.

'Incredible,' I said in awe. I couldn't even begin to work out how to build such a magnificent thing.

'He'd better not complain now,' said her dad as the last nail got hammered in. 'Right, luv, I'll see you later.' He winked and they all walked off as if dismantling and re-sizing an enormous structure was just one of those things you did in your lunch break.

'Amazing,' I whistled.

'Brilliant isn't it?' Jack grinned. 'I've been wanting to build something like this for years. Wish I hadn't needed help though, but never mind. Let's hope we don't get shouted at again by mad Roger, he's scary.'

'That's the least of our worries,' I replied as the three ponies came over to see if we had anything tasty in our pockets. 'She still hasn't moved them and I bet they'll still be here by the weekend.'

Jack sighed. 'Yes you're probably right. Well I'm too exhausted to think about it now. Let's just go with the flow.'

It was a sunny day on the Saturday of our move and Jack and I had a last look around to make sure we hadn't left anything at the yard.

'Right let's get those horses on-board!' came the shrill tones of Morag. She had a horsebox and had kindly offered to take our horses to the new field.

'Good boy, Buddy,' said Jack as he walked easily up the ramp and parked himself in the stall.

'Come on, Poppy, it's your turn now.' I walked nonchalantly towards the ramp and was feeling relieved that she was following me nicely. 'Oh God why have you stopped?' Poppy snorted and leaped sideways.

'Oh for God's sake,' I grumbled as I turned her around and tried again. 'Good girl,' I said with relief as she walked confidently up the ramp. 'Oh bloody hell, Poppy, why have you jumped off the bloody side?' Poppy snorted again and stamped her foot.

'What am I going to do?' I began to panic.

'I'll have a go,' laughed Jack and she took hold of the lead rope and tried to coax Poppy up the ramp. This time Poppy planted her feet halfway and refused to budge an inch. She wouldn't go forwards and she wouldn't go backwards.

'Oh goodness me,' said the flustered Morag. 'This is ridiculous, Poppy!'

'Do you need a hand?' Danny and Alex had arrived to wave us off. 'You pull and we'll push,' said Danny with a big grin.

I am ashamed to say that's what we did. I pulled on the rope while Jack, Danny and Alex pushed Poppy's big bottom and eventually we got her up the ramp.

'Morag, shall I give you some directions in case you lose us?' I asked.

'No time for that! I've got the address, just drive slowly in front of me!' Morag leaped into the driving seat and started the engine while Jack and I dashed to our respective cars.

It was a very strange feeling to look in my rear-view mirror and know that Poppy was in the horsebox behind me. All was going well until we came upon some road works. Morag got left behind and we couldn't pull in anywhere to wait for her. We just hoped that she would find her way. When I arrived at the field and opened the gate I noticed Jack had been up the day before and had created a fenced off carpark area. It was very impressive.

'You'd make someone a good husband,' I joked.

'Well if you can find me a wife that's not a total pain up the arse I might consider it. I keep attracting nutters,' replied Jack. 'I hope Morag isn't lost.'

We waited on the road so that she could see us.

'Shit, where is she?' I began to feel worried. More than fifteen minutes had passed.

'She's calling me,' Jack answered her phone. 'Hi Morag, are you ok?'

'Where are you?' shrieked Morag. Jack held the phone away from her ear and rubbed it.

'We're at the field. Where are you?'

'I'm in a pub carpark! I can't see you anywhere and the horses are getting very stressed! Where the hell are you?'

'Ok, Morag, calm down. I'll direct you,' replied Jack very calmly.

'Calm down? This is extremely stressful, Jacqueline. Your horses are going berserk back there!'

'Well let me direct you and they'll be ok when they get here. Are you at the Kite Inn?'

'Yes!'

'Great. Now can you come out of the carpark and turn left?'

All the while I could hear Morag huffing and puffing and becoming more and more loud and grumbling, but Jack kept her cool.

'Did you say turn right?' shouted Morag.

'No, turn left.'

'Oh hell's bells. I've gone the wrong way. Where the hell am I going to turn round?' Morag's voice yelled through the receiver.

'You'll see a farm yard coming up on your right, Morag, you can turn round in there,' replied Jack in her most soothing voice.

Morag huffed and puffed. Gears screeched, signalling that she was turning around.

'Ok, I'm coming back now. Where do I go next?'

'Great. Take the first left onto Village Road.'

'Oh yes I can see it now.'

'And then take the next right.'

'My goodness! I can't get my horse box down there it's nothing but a dirt track!' shouted Morag.

'You can easily get down there, Morag,' encouraged Jack.

'No I can't! Are you mad? I'll get stuck!'

'I absolutely promise you will not get stuck,' insisted Jack with calm authority.

'Oh my goodness! Oh my goodness!' We heard the engine accelerate. 'Oh yes, you're right. It's not so bad. Now where do I go?'

'Turn right and then after the bend you will see us in the road.' Jack mopped her brow and raised her eyebrows at me.

What a relief it was to see her drive round that bend and into our new carpark. Morag leaped out of the cab, red-faced and sweating profusely.

'Now we all need to put our riding hats and body protectors on before I open the ramp! This is highly dangerous, they are very very stressed!' instructed Morag with her eyes popping out.

'What? Are you serious?' I asked.

'Deadly serious!'

'Ok,' I replied, and dashed off to get my hat, as did Jack.

We all fastened our hats and hastily zipped up our body protectors ready for a rampage. Jack braced her legs and leaned slightly forwards with her arms outstretched, as if to catch a rugby ball. I felt sick with fear and hopped from one leg to another, dreading what sight would befall us. Morag slowly slid the bolts.

'Ok everyone, are you ready?' she asked, nervously.

'Yes!' we both replied. My heart was jumping into my mouth.

Morag tentatively let the ramp down and hurled herself out of harm's way. Poppy looked at us with disdain and sniffed the air delicately. Buddy was too busy devouring his haynet to bother to look round. Neither of them seemed remotely concerned.

'Oh,' I said as nothing happened.

'Ah, well they've obviously managed to calm themselves down, thank goodness,' said Morag looking slightly embarrassed.

'We all get flustered sometimes, Morag, it's ok.' Jack patted her on the back and walked up the ramp to untie Poppy.

Poppy sashayed down the ramp like a model on a catwalk and had a good look around while Jack had to drag Buddy away from his haynet. They walked around the field, sniffed about a bit and then put their heads down and began to graze as if they'd been there their whole lives.

'Well that was very boring,' laughed Jack. 'But it's great they're so relaxed.'

'Yes thank goodness for that,' agreed Morag. 'Now you girls take care and let us all know how you get on,' and with that she drove off.

'Where are the ponies?' I asked.

'Hiding over there,' Jack pointed into the back field where the three ponies were standing under a big oak tree. 'Weird. You'd have thought they'd come over wouldn't you?'

We hung around for a couple of hours to make sure everything was ok. The ponies finally came over and had a sniff of Poppy and Buddy, and then they all began to graze together, and as nothing in particular happened we realised it was safe to leave them.

'Thank goodness for that,' I said. 'I was worried that there might be a fight.'

'Yes, that's really lucky! Well let's leave them to settle in and meet tomorrow morning early.'

Chapter 9

Sunday morning arrived with a golden light tumbling through the bedroom window. It felt strange to be preparing to go to our own field and not the livery yard I had become accustomed to. The field was actually part of what had been a farm from pre-Edwardian times but it hadn't been worked for many years. The old farmhouse and outbuildings had all been renovated into a very posh house, which was a shame, but it still went by the name of Swallow Farm.

'Mummy, can I talk to you?' Florence was sitting on my bed, watching me pull my jodhpurs on. She was meant to be getting ready for a day out with Grandma and Grandad, which made me feel a bit guilty that I wasn't spending time with them yet once again expecting them to look after my daughter. They were such amazing parents and I knew they loved taking her out but I still felt a pang of selfishness. James was away on a course and I just wanted a day to myself.

'Of course you can talk to me.' I sat down next to Florence, wondering what was wrong.

'Lucia wasn't very nice to me this week and I don't know what to do,' Florence said sadly.

'Oh dear,' I took a sharp intake of breath as panic rose in my heart. 'What has she done?'

'She's been telling me that I can't play with her and Joanna and when I ask her why she just laughs and drags Joanna away.'

'That's not very nice.' I wanted to use other words but managed to control the urge. 'What did you do?'

'I went to sit on a bench,' replied Florence sadly.

'Was that every playtime?' I was enraged and heartbroken for my daughter and had to work hard to appear calm.

'Yes.'

'Was there no one else you could play with?'

'I didn't want to ask anyone else.'

'Why ever not?' I did my best to keep my voice level.

'I didn't want anyone else to say I couldn't play,' Florence rubbed her eyes. I swallowed and tried to work out what I could say that would be helpful. What I wanted to say might not have been very constructive.

'Friday was a bit better,' said Florence.

'What happened on Friday?'

'Another girl asked me to play.'

'Well that's very nice. And is she kind, this other girl?'

'Yes. We had a nice time skipping.'

'Well that's really good. She sounds lovely,' I said with relief. 'Do you think you need to be friends with Lucia?'

Florence looked thoughtful. 'No I don't.'

'I agree. Why don't you invite your new friend for tea after school next week?'

'That's a good idea, thank you, Mummy.' Florence smiled and skipped away to get ready for her day out.

I took a deep breath as memories of my own childhood surfaced. Girls can be so nasty. I was relieved that Florence had made a new friend but felt worried that she might be as sensitive as I had been.

What a little bitch! I shouted in my head. *She needs a slap! But what can I do to help strengthen Flo? Karate? Judo?*

My phone rang and interrupted my pondering.

'You'd better come quick! Poppy's been injured!' shouted Jack as soon as I answered. 'One of those bloody ponies kicked her and it looks pretty bad.'

I felt sick and my heart began to race. Fortunately, my parents arrived to collect Florence so I left them to it and dashed out of the house. Luckily it was only a five-minute drive to our field but it felt like it took forever to get there and I dreaded what I would find when I arrived. I screeched to a halt in the carpark and hurled myself out of the door with such force I fell over. Jack's dad was there and he ran over to pick me up.

'Don't worry, luv. I've cleaned it up and sprayed it with purple spray,' he said as he pulled me to my feet. Poppy was standing nearby with a big cut on her leg, which Jack's dad had expertly cleaned up.

'I were a stock man years ago so I know my way around a wounded animal. She'll be right in a few days but keep spraying this on to keep it clean.' He handed me a tin of iodine spray and I thanked him profusely. 'You'll have to get rid o' them beasts. They're a menace. We've made a separate paddock to keep 'em away from your two but they can't stay in there for long.' He shook his head and got into his car and drove away.

'That was so lucky your dad knew what to do!' I said.

'Yes, he's great with cows. I suppose a horse isn't much different,' said Jack. 'But he's right. We can't have these ponies causing so much trouble, especially when the owner isn't even paying her rent! What shall we do?'

'I'm so annoyed about Poppy's leg. I want to move them!'

'Move them?' asked Jack.

'Yes, move them to another field. That bloody woman is taking the piss and I have lost my patience! I've been calling her and texting her all week and she won't reply. We're going to walk them to that field next to Valerie's yard right now!' I was so upset about Poppy's leg.

'Wow! Ok, good idea. But I think we need to wait till lunchtime or Valerie will see us,' said Jack, practical as ever. 'And we need a third person to help us.'

'Oh God yes. But who?'

'How about that woman on the black horse? I bet she'd help. She can't stand Anna.'

'Great idea! Let's bob round there now and see if we can find her,' I suggested.

We jumped into Jack's van and drove the very short distance to the farm opposite the pub and luckily the lady was in the yard, grooming her horse in the sun. It was a stunning animal and reminded me of the toy Sindy horse I'd had when I was a child.

'Hello!' she said with surprise when we got out of the van.

'Hi. We didn't get your name the other day,' I replied. 'I'm Grace and this is Jack.'

'I'm Sapna and this is Velvet.' She patted her beautiful horse. 'Did you come to look at the yard? There are two stables available I believe.'

'Oh no, we're not moving,' I replied.

'Don't blame you, this road is way too busy. I wish I was still over where you are,' she sighed wistfully.

'We actually came to ask a favour. Would you be up for helping us move those ponies?' I asked. 'One of them kicked Poppy and she's got a pretty bad cut on her leg so I've lost my patience with Anna now.'

'Oh no! Was it the bay?' asked Sapna.

'Yes it was,' said Jack. 'How did you know?'

'She regularly kicked and bit Velvet, which is another reason why I left. She had two black ponies when I was there and they were really nippy too,' replied Sapna. 'Lucky there's only the three there now. Where do you want to move them to?'

'There's a field that we know is empty and it's about a half-hour walk from here. Would you help us to lead them there?' I asked.

'Yes, absolutely. It would be a pleasure to help. Anna needs to be shown that people won't put up with her behaviour. When do you want to do it?'

'I think we should set off at twelve. Hopefully there won't be much traffic at lunchtime,' said Jack. 'Can you come to our field?'

'Will do. And I've got a few headcollars I'll bring if you need them.'

'Brilliant, thank you,' I said. 'I'd not thought of that.'

'No worries. See you at the field at twelve.' Sapna grinned.

'I can't believe we're doing this,' said Jack as we drove back to the field. 'I hope we don't get done by the police or anything?'

'Right now, I really don't care,' I replied.

'Ok let's sort out the practicalities. First, we need to take a big bucket over there and loads of water. We'll take it in my van, which we'll leave there so we can drive afterwards so you'll have to follow me in your car. And we need a new chain and a number padlock so they're safe in the field. We'll give her the number obviously.' Jack thought of everything.

We went straight to the shops to buy what we needed and filled a massive container with water, which weighed a ton. Then we drove to the overgrown field.

'This is the maddest thing I've ever done,' said Jack as we sneaked down the bridle path to find the gate into the overgrown field. 'Thank God the grass is so tall. Valerie shouldn't be able to see us. Shit get down! She's there!' We dived to the ground.

'Where was she? I didn't see her!' I whispered.

'She was in her field doing something with Siegmund!' Jack whispered back. 'That's all we need, bloody Valerie seeing us now.'

'What shall we do?'

'We'll have to crawl,' hissed Jack. I don't know why we were whispering because Valerie was far enough away but it always felt as if she could hear everything for miles around her. We scooted along on all fours, dragging the water container and large bucket and waited at the gate for about ten minutes until we felt brave enough to check if Valerie was still there or not.

'She's gone!' we both said in unison.

'Quick! Let's get this stuff in the field and get out of here before she comes back,' gasped Jack and we hurriedly did the deed and scampered back down the bridle path.

'Good job nobody's out here riding,' I said. 'Where are you going to leave your van?'

'We'll park it up that lane near the farm. Nobody will see it and we can get to it easily after we've dropped the ponies.'

We drove back to the field in my car, feeling like the Guy Fawkes conspirators.

'I feel a bit nervous now,' I admitted. 'Is it awful to do this?'

'I don't think so, no,' replied Jack thoughtfully. 'The owner is taking the total piss and her pony has injured Poppy. And don't forget it also injured Sapna's horse so I think realistically we are not in the wrong for removing them.'

'Yes, I just hope we don't get arrested.'

'I'm sure we won't,' said Jack. 'Right, what time is it? How long have we got till D-Day?' I looked at my watch and it was almost time. My stomach felt full of butterflies now that my idea was almost becoming reality. I felt sorry for the ponies for having such a weird owner and I hoped that Sapna was right and that Anna did have other fields to take them to.

'Hello,' greeted Sapna with a big grin as she walked into our carpark. 'Are you ready? It's so exciting to do this! Anna is such a cow.'

'I hope we can get headcollars on them,' replied Jack, looking over to where the ponies were grazing. 'My dad got them into a small paddock so shouldn't be too hard to catch them.'

'They're pretty good, I've had to handle them a few times so I'm sure it'll be fine,' said Sapna, handing us each a headcollar and lead rope. With trepidation, we walked across to the ponies and thankfully they were all easy to catch.

'Ok ladies, I've worked out a route that avoids most of the main roads so I'll go in front,' said Jack. Sapna and I arranged ourselves behind.

Luckily, it was a nice sunny and still day so the ponies were very relaxed as we walked down the lane. It was a great opportunity to see part of the village I hadn't ventured into before. The old Edwardian schoolhouse had been renovated into a family home and so had the old village hall. In the woods, the remains of the old church lay scattered amongst fallen trees but interestingly there were no gravestones so they must have buried people elsewhere. Eventually, we passed the main farm house which was still a working farm. Rolling fields spread out all around like a patchwork quilt of various crops just beginning to grow and through the pine trees the reservoir was sparkling and looked for all the world like a Scottish loch. The hedges were busy with little birds tweeting, busily building nests, and thankfully the roads were quiet and the walk didn't take as long as we had expected.

'Thank God, nobody's around,' said Jack as we walked past Valerie's yard. 'Let's get them in that field quick!' We led the ponies down the bridle path, opened the gate and led them in. We showed them where the water was and then turned them loose. The ponies were not in the least perturbed and began grazing very happily despite the grass being so incredibly tall and old and full of monstrous weeds.

'Phew!' we all said together.

'What now?' asked Sapna.

'I think we should all get in my van and then Grace you can text Anna and tell her what we've done. Actually, let's take a photo so she can see they're ok,' replied Jack. I took a photo on my phone and then we all legged it to the van, which was parked on a lane by the farm opposite. It was higher up than the field so we had a very good view.

'Hi Anna,' I read aloud as I texted. 'As you have not replied to any of my calls and have not moved your ponies, we have removed them from the field. They are safe. Here is a photo and the exact location.' I sent her a Google Maps screenshot so she knew exactly where they were. We waited with bated breath for over fifteen very long minutes.

'Oh my God she's replied!' My heart leaped.

'What's she said?' asked Jack and Sapna together.

'You absolute bitch!' I read out. 'How could you do that when you know I have no money and my daughter is sick in hospital?'

'What daughter?' laughed Sapna. 'She hasn't got kids!'

'You don't have children,' I replied. Then my phone rang.

'Oh shit. It's the landlord!' I squeaked.

'What the hell have you done?' he bellowed down the phone, so loud I had to hold it away from my ear. 'I've had Anna on the phone crying! She said you've taken her ponies somewhere and you won't tell her where! Her son's in hospital on kidney dialysis! Bring those ponies back this instant or the police will be involved!' I felt sick. Sapna grabbed the phone.

'Hi Roger, it's me, Sapna,' she said.

'Sapna? What the hell are you doing there? Don't tell me you're involved? You're all gonna end up in prison for this!' he shouted.

'No we aren't,' replied Sapna very calmly. 'Anna doesn't have any children and she has other fields all over the place which she also doesn't pay for. She knows exactly where these ponies are so there is no problem. She is also a very wealthy woman. She is winding you up!'

'You're kidding?' said Roger, clearly flabbergasted.

'No I am not kidding. She is taking the piss out of you. I did try to tell you ages ago.'

'Oh right. Silly bitch. Carry on,' and he hung up.

'Wow! I thought we were in for it,' laughed Jack. My phone rang again. This time it was a withheld number.

'Answer it! It might be Anna,' said Jack. So I tentatively answered and put it on loudspeaker.

'Is that Grace?' said a man's voice.

'Yes. Who are you?' I replied.

'I'm Police Constable Jefferies from West Yorkshire Police.

We've had a report that you've stolen three ponies from a field. This is a serious allegation. The owner is extremely distressed and has a son in hospital awaiting a liver transplant. You are causing her a great deal of upset, Mrs Olson. Can you tell me what's going on?'

Jack and Sapna opened their mouths in shock and I had no idea what to say.

'Have you stolen the ponies, Mrs Olson?' asked the policeman. I sprang back to life.

'No I have not stolen them! And in fact I am extremely annoyed! We have removed the ponies because she has not been paying her rent and we gave her enough notice to quit. Also she does not have any children. She is a compulsive liar! We have told her exactly where they are and have even given her a Google Maps screenshot so she can come and get them whenever she likes.'

'Right. Well this sounds a bit more complex. Can you tell me where you are so we can come and talk to you, Mrs Olson?'

'Oh my God are you serious?' I couldn't believe my ears.

'I'm always serious, Mrs Olson,' replied the policeman, so I told him where we were and we waited. Jack burst out laughing from the shock and Sapna just grinned inanely.

'Haven't you got a solicitor in your family?' asked Jack, suddenly being practical again. 'Call her now!'

'Oh hell yes! It's my cousin Robyn. She lives there!' I pointed to a large white house, next to the farm. My cousin and I had spent many happy hours together when we were younger milking the cows at the farm, and Robyn still lived there with her now elderly parents.

'Come on,' said Jack, jumping out of her van and running to the door. Thankfully Robyn was in.

'Robyn help!' I shouted. 'I'm about to get arrested!'

'You bloody idiot,' laughed Robyn. 'What on earth have you done?' I poured out the entire story. 'Right, I'll get my work clothes on and I'll come and talk to the police.'

'This is like a tv show,' laughed Jack. Five minutes later, the police car rolled up.

'Hello ladies, I'm here to ask you about the ponies,' said the policeman very seriously.

'Good afternoon, Officer, I am Mrs Olson's solicitor,' said my cousin Robyn, stepping out of her front door.

'Solicitor? I'm sure there's no need for that,' said the slightly stunned policeman.

'Well I'm here now,' replied Robyn and she took my phone and handed it to the policeman. 'As you can see, my client has been very clear with the owner. She has given her enough warning to remove her ponies and she has also given her a photograph and very clear directions as to where the ponies are. Is this a theft?'

The policeman read through all the texts and looked very annoyed. 'No it's not a theft it's a big waste of police time. I've got more important things to do than this!' Without another word he stomped off angrily and got into his car and drove away.

'Wow. Thank you so much for doing that, Robyn,' I gasped.

'No problem. I was actually about to go out for the day so you were lucky to catch me,' Robyn laughed. 'I knew you wouldn't get arrested for this, it's just a load of rubbish. She sounds like a right pain in the arse!'

'She is.' Sapna nodded her head.

'Well I'd better get going. See you later and stay out of trouble.'

Robyn winked and went back into her house to change out of her work clothes.

'Christ, this is turning into a soap opera! Look here comes a horse box,' Jack hopped from one foot to the other with excitement. We all squatted down and peeped through the hedge so that Anna couldn't see us. The horsebox was almost new and big enough for four large horses.

'No money?' said Jack.

'I told you she's a liar,' replied Sapna.

We watched as Anna got out of the cab and called her ponies. They all trotted over to her. She put headcollars on them and led them up the ramp of her very posh horsebox.

'Let's follow her!' suggested Jack.

'Ooh yes!' I agreed and we leaped into the van and surreptitiously followed Anna at a distance. Ten minutes later, Anna pulled onto a dirt track which led to a farm. We parked in a layby and then we followed on foot and hid behind a very handy old shed. She led the ponies to a field which had two black ponies in. 'Those are the ponies I told you about,' hissed Sapna.

As Anna turned the ponies into the large field, Jack took several photos as well as a photo of her getting back into her horsebox. We waited for her to drive away and then we got back into Jack's van.

'Well,' said Jack, with a big grin on her face. 'I think that was a success.'

'I've got another text,' I said as my phone pinged. 'It's from Anna!'

'Read it out!' said Sapna excitedly.

'Ha! She says, "You will be hearing from the police for stealing my ponies. You know I have no money to pay for transport to move them and I am in hospital with my very sick daughter. What you have done is evil." Oh my God she's such a liar!' I couldn't believe what she'd just sent me.

'She's thick as pig shit isn't she?' said Jack. 'Isn't it obvious that we would have been waiting and watching all of this? Send her the photos I took. Let's see what she says.' Jack sent me the photos to send over to Anna.

'You will be hearing from the police about wasting their time and here is the evidence,' I read out loud as I typed. 'There now, let's see what she says to that.'

After a while of no response it was obvious that Anna had realised she had finally been beaten. We drove back to the field, very hyped up from the day's adventure.

'Thank you for the fun,' chuckled Sapna as we dropped her back at her farm. 'Do you fancy meeting for a hack? It would be nice to have some company for a change. Nobody else rides much from here.'

'Yes, that would be great,' I replied. 'We have no idea where to ride round here.'

'I'll show you some good places to go. There are loads of beautiful rides,' said Sapna. We arranged a date and set off to check on our horses.

All was peaceful in the field and Poppy's cut looked a bit better than it had done so that was a relief.

'I'm going home to get into a nice hot bubble bath,' sighed Jack. 'I think I've earned it.'

'That's a good idea. I might have to do the same, my nerves are jangling after all that. I thought we were in serious trouble!'

'Me too. Thank God for your cousin saving our backsides,' laughed Jack.

As I drove away, I felt a mixture of sorrow for the ponies who had to put up with such a weird owner and triumph for having done something so extremely out of the ordinary. I also thanked God profusely for providing me with a cousin who was a solicitor.

Oh hell, what to do about Florence though? My mind went back to the conversation we'd had earlier. *I don't want her to end up like me.*

My heart dropped into my boots at the thought of her experiencing what I had. Every morning, the whole journey to school had been filled with dread. I still remember the misery washing over me as my mum's car would turn into the long driveway that led into the carpark. How I had forced myself to swallow my fears and pretend I was ok. I didn't want Florence to be like that and I was glad she had been able to talk to me. To this day I still don't know why I hid the truth from my parents.

Chapter 10

Monday began in a quiet sort of a way. Florence didn't seem perturbed about going to school, in fact she was looking forward to inviting her new friend over for tea, so that was a relief. I wasn't working until later so I was able to go up to the field to check on Poppy's wound. It was healing well but I didn't want to ride her until it was properly scabbed over. It was then that reality hit me in the face.

Crikey! How many poos do they do? Oh hell. I've never had to do this before. What a pain in the arse. I don't have time for extra jobs like this, I really should be seeing my mum. I'm such a terrible daughter.

I sighed and pondered on my new sense of guilt around my mum. Since she had retired, I felt that I should do more with her yet she was very happy going out for day trips with my dad so I couldn't really understand why my mind kept prodding me about it. I told myself to shut up. Jack had bought some new wheelbarrows and poop scoopers and now it was time to christen them.

'I didn't realise how much poo they did,' I complained as Jack walked into the field.

'I read an article that said a horse does about eighteen turds a day,' replied Jack. 'So we'll soon get rid of our bingo wings! And it will need clearing regularly or the grass will get nasty. To be honest I thought you'd be too much of a princess to do this. I'm amazed to see you with a shit shovel in your hand, you look so funny,' she roared with laughter.

'A princess?' I was very offended. 'I don't think so. Anyway, even if I was there's only you and me to do it so I shall crack on if you don't mind.' Jack laughed again and grabbed a scoop and rake. We both had the field cleared quite quickly as we worked together and it certainly was good exercise. But it stressed me out to think that it was now a new daily chore.

'Right. I'd better get going. I'll wait to ride with you when Poppy's leg's all sorted. My dad wants to go to the auction today to look at cows. He's obsessed with them. What are you up to?' asked Jack.

'I'm working and then I'm taking Florence to a new riding school. The other place was awful. They kept hitting the ponies and Florence got really upset and wanted to give up riding. So hopefully this place will be nicer.'

'Have fun,' Jack winked and we both left the field.

Florence's new riding school was actually not that far from our field, in a very posh village called Bramhope.

'Think Like a Pony,' said Florence, reading the sign as we drove into the car park. 'That's a funny name isn't it, Mummy?'

'Yes, I suppose it is. I wonder what it means? I'm sure we'll soon find out.' I stepped out of the car and looked around. There was a very beautiful Yorkshire stone farmhouse with large, well-maintained stone barns, surrounded by glorious green fields that were just beginning to bloom like ours. The outdoor arena, with its black rubber surface, was very impressive and everything looked very new and clean. I hadn't realised how filthy the previous riding school had been until I set eyes on Think Like a Pony.

'Hello, you must be Florence?' greeted a very cheery voice. I looked round to see a very smiley faced young woman leading a small chocolate brown New Forest pony. 'I'm Alice and this is Conker. Let's go into the outdoor arena as it's nice and sunny today.' We followed Alice over to the perfect arena where in a far corner another child was having a lesson on a little grey pony.

'We start all the kids off one to one here so that we can ensure the ponies are comfortable and the kids are safe,' explained Alice. I was very pleased to hear both of those sentiments as the previous place was not that considerate. 'Mum can stay here and watch over the fence while we go in and get started, ok Florence?'

Florence nodded and followed Alice and Conker into the arena while I sat down on a chair near the fence.

'I know you've ridden before but let's start at the very beginning, greeting the pony,' Alice smiled and Florence looked very serious. 'Now, did you know that ponies are very clever animals? They have super senses!'

Florence shook her head and replied, 'We weren't taught very well at the other place. They weren't very nice to the ponies.'

'Oh dear,' Alice tutted. 'Well, we love all our ponies and we're going to teach you how to hear what they are saying. Do you like the sound of that?'

'Yes,' Florence nodded and smiled shyly.

'Great stuff. Well first of all we have to make sure that these lovely ponies are as happy to be ridden as we are to ride them,' Alice continued. 'So, let's start by saying "Hello" and to do that we take a deep breath. Can you do that?' Florence took a very deep breath.

'Lovely. Now let's roll our shoulders and make sure there's no tension,' Alice demonstrated and Florence copied. 'Excellent. Now that we are relaxed that will help Conker to feel relaxed too.

So the next thing is to take a gentle step forwards and put your hand on his shoulder.'

Florence stepped towards Conker and put her hand on his shoulder. He curved his head round and put his nose on her cheek and had a good sniff.

'Ah, that's lovely,' said Alice enthusiastically. 'Conker's saying, "Hello! I'm very pleased to meet you!" Isn't that nice?' Florence nodded. 'So now that Conker has said hello, let's walk around the arena with him so you can both get to know each other.' Florence's face fell and she took a step backwards.

'What's wrong, Florence?' asked Alice kindly.

'He might not want to be friends with me,' she mumbled, her cheeks flushing red.

My heart felt like it paused and I didn't know whether to get up and say something or keep out of the way.

'What's made you think about that?' Alice asked gently.

'Well, Lucia doesn't want me to play with them any more so it must be something I've done.'

My mouth dropped open with horror and I jumped to my feet. Alice put her hand up and shook her head, indicating I should stay still.

'Do you believe that you've done anything wrong?' Alice sat down on a nearby mounting block so that she was at eye level with Florence while Conker stood quietly.

Florence looked like she was thinking very deeply and eventually shook her head.

'No. I haven't done anything,' she concluded.

'Well that's good.' Alice smiled. 'If you know, deep in your heart that you have done nothing, whose problem is this?'

'It's Lucia's,' replied Florence.

'Absolutely right, Florence. It sounds to me that Lucia is choosing to be unkind. Is that how we should treat our friends?'

'No.' Florence shook her head.

'Exactly. We should be kind. And if someone is being unkind then they are not people that we want to be near. You know, if you were an unkind person, Conker wouldn't have given you a big sniff. He would have walked away. Look at him now, where has he wandered to?'

'To me.' Florence smiled as she noticed that Conker was standing right next to her.

'That's his way of saying he wants to be your friend, and he only does that to nice people.' Alice grinned widely. 'Shall we go for a walk with him?'

Florence grinned back and nodded her head and off they went round the arena together with Alice just far enough away so that she wasn't intruding on the bonding between them.

'Ok that's great.' Alice smiled as they came to a halt near me. 'I'm very proud that Florence was able to talk so clearly about her feelings about Lucia. And Conker has helped her to see that she herself is a lovely girl.' I choked back tears and nodded. Florence looked very happy.

'Now it's time to mount,' said Alice as she turned back to me and said, 'As you can see, we like all our students to start on a lead rein first as this helps them to get an understanding of how the ponies move in a controlled environment. It also enables them to develop true balance and an independent seat. This way, the children are much safer riders and they don't pull on the pony's mouth.'

'Excellent,' I nodded. It all sounded fascinating to me.

Alice led Conker to the mounting block and Florence got herself on. It was wonderful to see the attention to detail regarding correct hand and leg position and I learned a lot just from watching. Florence had a big grin on her face and it was such a relief to see her passion for riding had been reignited.

'That's all for today, Florence, so off you get and let's give Conker a big cuddle to say thank you.' Florence leaned forwards and gave him a big hug round his neck. Then she jumped off and gave him a kiss.

'Thank you,' I said to Alice. 'That was all absolutely incredible. I'm lost for words!'

'You're very welcome. Look forward to seeing you again next weekend.' Alice smiled and led Conker away and we walked back to the car.

'Did you enjoy it?' I asked.

'Yes, it was really fun.' Florence grinned. 'I love Conker.'

'Conker's my favourite pony,' said a voice behind me, which made me startle. 'He was the first pony I rescued for my riding school.' I turned to see who was talking and found that it was a lady of indeterminate age but older than me. She was small and wiry and had a very warm smile.

'I'm Lynn,' she greeted with a firm handshake. 'And you must be Grace and Florence?'

'Yes, we are. I'm very impressed that you know our names,' I replied.

'I like to get to know everyone who comes here because I feel it's so important for the growth of each child.'

'That's a great ethos,' I said. 'I'm blown away by what just happened in the lesson. It was so different to how it was for me when I was learning to ride. It was all about just staying on, really,' I laughed. 'It certainly didn't include any emotional exploration.'

'Yes, nobody ever really considered anything more than that did they?' agreed Lynn. 'Would you like to come and meet the rest of the ponies, Florence? I'm just on my way to check on them now and you can help.' Florence smiled and nodded.

We followed Lynn down a path behind the carpark which led to a lovely airy open-sided structure. Inside there were stalls where the ponies were having a snooze. All around were beautiful green fields as far as the eye could see.

'Every day we bring them in for a few hours of loafing in between lessons,' explained Lynn. 'We like them to be fully rested and relaxed so that they're safe when they're with the children. The rest of the time they've got free roam of all our lovely grassland. Aren't they lucky?' They were indeed very lucky as it was such a beautiful and natural meadow with various trees just coming into leaf for shelter and a wide stream.

'I'd love to know more about how the lessons will unfold,' I said as Florence wandered off to stroke a lovely little chestnut pony. 'It seems such an unusual approach. Alice really helped Florence just now with a bullying issue at school.'

'That's what we love to do here,' replied Lynn, absently stroking a pony. 'Riding is just a part of it. I believe that humans are drawn to horses because it leads to healing. There's something unique about the horse that seems to facilitate change.'

'Well what I just saw Alice do with Florence amazed me.'

'It is amazing, isn't it?'

'How did you get into this way of teaching? It's astonishing.'

'Well it was actually an accident. I was never interested in horses but a doctor suggested we get a pony to help our son with some issues he was dealing with. I liked the idea and we had all this land doing nothing so I had to learn to ride too but I didn't like the methods they used at the riding school. So I ended up in America learning from some of the natural horsemanship teachers and that led to me developing my own teaching programme. I had experience of being a schoolteacher already, which helped.'

'How fantastic.' I nodded. 'It's so lovely to hear how much you care about all of these ponies. Did you say that Conker was a rescue?'

'Yes, I'm very happy to say that all these ponies are rescued from neglect and in some cases abuse. I've trained them all myself and they're cracking little riding school ponies now.' Lynn smiled proudly.

'Wow, that's brilliant.' I was very impressed.

'You can achieve anything with love, kindness and clear boundaries,' she replied. 'It's very simple really. And that's what we'll be teaching Florence. We work with a lot of kids who have been excluded from school. Some of our work here is all about teaching youngsters self-respect and how to speak up for themselves so they can go and get good jobs and have a better life. The lady who taught Florence today was actually on her way to prison when she first came here. The work we did with her has changed her life completely.' Lynn grinned.

'No way,' I gasped.

'Horses are the best teachers.' Lynn winked. 'You'll see as you watch Florence in her lessons how we subtly introduce the concepts of self-respect, self-discipline, boundaries, love and kindness. All the things we need to succeed in life. If she's being bullied at school, she won't be for much longer, I can promise you that.'

By this point, I was so overcome with the wonderfulness of it all that I choked up. What a truly remarkable thing to have accidentally stumbled upon such a transformative place. I coughed and smiled, trying to stop myself from crying. My heart felt like it was bursting out of my chest and up into my throat and I wished that I could have lessons there too. Sadly, we could only afford Florence's lessons but I was determined to learn as much as I could by just watching.

I was spared the need to say anything more because just at that moment, one of the instructors came along and needed to get some advice from Lynn so it was a good opportunity to leave and pull myself together. As the riding school was so close to our field, Florence and I popped in to check on Poppy's wound.

'I'm going to practise saying hello properly to Poppy,' said Florence enthusiastically.

'What a good idea,' I replied. 'You have a go and let's see what happens.'

Poppy and Buddy wandered over to greet us and Florence took a deep breath, wriggled her shoulders and then stepped forwards to reach her hand up onto Poppy's shoulder, which was a lot higher up than Conker's. 'Hello Poppy,' she said as Poppy sniffed the top of her head. 'Aww! She's saying hello to me, Mummy.'

'Ah yes, how lovely. One day you'll be big enough to ride her too.' I smiled. 'Can you check on her cut while you're close to it?' Florence looked very pleased to have been asked to check on something important and I was very relieved to see it was still improving.

We spent a while just chatting to Buddy and Poppy and then we went home. Florence wanted to do some clay modelling, which gave me the chance to sit down and think about all that had happened during the riding lesson. Think Like a Pony had made such a deep impression so I had a look at their fascinating website. It was very absorbing to read all about their transformative methods. It blew my mind to think how perfect this place was for Florence and I had only booked her in because my mum had spotted it on the way back from a garden centre. I couldn't wait to see what would happen in Florence's next lesson.

Chapter 11

The drive to school the following day was filled with mixed emotions. I wondered if the experience at Think Like a Pony would help Florence to feel differently about the situation with Lucia. She had said nothing more about it, but even so, I had secretly phoned school to tell them what had been happening and they said they would keep an eye on things, which eased my mind a little.

Why are girls so nasty? I pondered inwardly. *What is it about certain people that attract the horribleness of a bully? Was I just too soft? Why couldn't I stick up for myself? She never bothered anyone else. I really hope Florence will be ok now.*

The week zipped past and fortunately nothing was mentioned about Lucia. Florence seemed to be enjoying herself with her new friend so I got swallowed up in a blur of work, shit shovelling, wound care, dog training, mum stuff, feeling guilty about not seeing enough of my own mum and mountains of housework. But then time seemed to suddenly pause on Friday, which was wonderful because I had a day off and my parents were out on a daytrip. After depositing Florence at school and walking Wrexford in the woods, I took a moment to breathe and relax.

There's a whole pile of washing to do and I need to sew those new curtains. The inner drudge sneaked its way into my consciousness.

Sod off! It's Friday I am absolutely not doing any of that rubbish! A new rebellious voice came through, which pleased me greatly. I suddenly felt the way I had when I was a teenager and used to bunk off school to go and eat ring doughnuts at Sainsbury's. It was so naughty but so fun. Jack and I had arranged to meet Sapna for a ride so chores were going to have to wait. I leaped into the car full of excitement about discovering new places to ride. The sky was blue and the trees were covered in more leaves and the best thing was, it only took five minutes to reach the field as opposed to fifteen minutes to get to the old yard.

'Take cover!' yelled Jack as I stepped out of my car. Jack dived to the ground next to her van as I heard a strange pinging noise close to my ear.

'What's that noise?' I asked.

'Get down!' she shouted. Ping! Ping! Ping! In the distance I could hear banging. 'It's shotgun pellets!'

'Ow! Bloody hell! What the heck?' Something had hit my shoulder.

'Field shelter! Quick!' Jack ran towards the gate that led into the field. 'Bollocks!' Somehow, her sleeve got caught on the gate post and she fell face down with a thud. I pulled her to her feet and we dashed into the shelter.

'What the hell is going on?' I peeped out of the shelter to try to see what was happening.

'Dunno! But if my van's damaged, I'll be furious.'

Suddenly the banging stopped and we tentatively stepped out into the field. Both horses were trotting around, clearly upset by the whole thing but they calmed down quite quickly.

'I can do without that on a Friday morning,' I grumbled, rubbing my shoulder.

'On any morning,' agreed Jack. 'Hope they've finished now. Let's have a look at you.' Jack pulled my top open and peered at my shoulder. 'Can't see anything. Must be just like an air rifle pellet from a distance maybe?'

'Let's get tacked up and get out of here before it starts again!' I suggested.

'Yeah good plan.'

Luckily it remained quiet as we groomed and tacked up and then I noticed a large wooden mounting block in the carpark.

'What do you think?' asked Jack proudly. 'I made it out of my neighbour's old decking wood that he was chucking out.'

'It's brilliant!' I was very impressed. 'I wouldn't have a clue how to do any of that stuff.'

'I think you might have to learn now that it's just us up here. I'll give you a few lessons.' Jack grinned. My heart sank at the reminder of how much responsibility we had taken on by moving our horses away from the safety of a livery yard to our own field. Jack had been born with a hammer in her hand. She really was so talented at joinery, it was always fascinating to see the things she could make. I, on the other hand, had absolutely no idea whatsoever about that sort of thing and doubted I could learn.

'Morning!' greeted the cheery voice of Sapna as she appeared at our gate on her beautiful horse. 'Are you ready to explore?'

'Yes!' said Jack and I simultaneously. It was very exciting and all thoughts of field maintenance melted away.

'I thought I'd show you a nice circular route around the farm today. It's an easy ride and will take about an hour. How does that sound?'

'Anything sounds great,' said Jack enthusiastically. We mounted and took the first steps out of the field.

The lane wound round a bend, over a little bridge with woods on the left and Valentina's old stone farmhouse on the right. A stream bubbled through the woods next to the remains of the derelict brick church. It was very small and I wondered what life had been like for the people who had lived in the village hundreds of years ago. Then the lane led us round to a very big farmhouse and acres of fields opened up on both sides.

'The farmer's lovely but the old guy who works for him can be a bit funny so watch out for him,' warned Sapna.

'In what way funny?' I asked, intrigued.

'You're about to find out,' she replied as a large blue tractor appeared on the lane ahead. 'Quick! We've got to hurry!' She urged her horse into a trot and we did the same not knowing what was happening.

'Is he not going to stop?' I couldn't believe the speed at which he was approaching us.

'Jesus, is he mental?' yelled Jack.

'Turn here!' shouted Sapna and we all three turned off the lane onto the bridle path with only moments to spare before the tractor thundered past.

'What a horrible man!' I gasped, patting Poppy for being so brave. 'And weird! His face was expressionless. How creepy.'

'Yeah, he's very odd. His face is always the same.' Sapna nodded. 'Anyway, you can always hear him coming, which is sort of helpful.'

I felt very uncomfortable about a crazy man in a tractor who could potentially kill me but I began to relax as we walked down the bridle path that took us round the back of the farm. All around were beautiful rolling fields. Some were dotted with blobs of fluffy cotton-wool sheep and some were showing the first signs of crops.

The hedgerow on either side of the path was brimming with life as little birds flitted in and out. It was absolutely glorious and I breathed in the scent of fresh pine.

'For goodness' sake, Daphne, will you stand still?' shrilled a posh lady's voice from round a bend in the path. 'Hang on!' she called out to us as we came to a stop behind her. 'I can't tolerate this inconvenience any longer.'

The voice belonged to a woman on a large bay thoroughbred. She was standing up in her stirrups, trimming the over-hanging branches of a gnarled and ancient oak tree using a pair of shears. Her horse stood very quietly as all the cuttings cascaded onto her back and bounced onto the ground. The three of us watched, open mouthed at the bizarre spectacle.

'Damn it. I knew I should have brought the chainsaw. I can't get any more off. Never mind! It's better than it was.' She sat back down in the saddle and turned her horse around to greet us. She looked to be at least sixty-five years old and ready for a round of golf in her pale pink corduroys and lemon sweater with pale blue diamond pattern. Instead of a riding hat she wore a head scarf emblazoned with orange roses. 'Oh hello! I'm Gillian. We own the farm over there.' She waved her arm, gesturing to a non-specific location.

We each introduced ourselves and said where our horses lived.

'Ah!' she said when we told her where our field was. 'Now Valentina is lovely but her husband can be quite fierce, so beware of him.' She nodded knowingly. 'Are you headed in this direction? I'll ride with you if you are.'

Gillian seemed to have a wealth of local knowledge as she regaled us with comical tales of rides she'd been on with various people from the area over the years. It turned out she had bred the horse she was riding as her hobby was thoroughbreds.

'Your mare looks like a thoroughbred to me,' she said pointing at Poppy.

'She's an Irish sports horse,' I replied. 'Or at least that's what it says on her passport.'

'Rubbish!' Gillian trilled. 'That's a thoroughbred or I don't know my bacon!'

I could almost hear Jack smirking and wondered what she was going to say but I didn't have time to wonder for long. Bang! Bang! Bang! came the sound of shotguns. All the horses started snorting and prancing around. In the distance I could see a group of men lying down with guns pointing up at the sky. My heart began thumping like a drum.

'Oh for the love of God. Not this again!' said Gillian, exasperated.

'Should we turn back?' I asked hopefully.

'No! We shall not be defeated,' declared Gillian.

'If we turn round, the horses are more likely to bolt,' said Sapna with what sounded like experience.

'Great! Let's ride straight into the war zone,' said Jack. Sadly, her sarcasm was lost on Gillian.

'Excellent attitude! Daphne's an old hand at this lark,' she replied, gathering her reins and urging her horse onwards. 'Come along, Daphne! Walk on!'

The gunshots started up again and Poppy began snorting and jogging. I felt an overwhelming desire to vomit. Although we could hear the tirade of shots, there was nothing falling from the sky.

'They rarely hit anything!' shouted Sapna above the din. 'They're a bunch of daft old men who have nothing better to do than try to shoot pigeons and crows! I don't think they can see very well either.' That last comment filled me with horror.

Oh my God! If they can't see they might hit us! I worried silently.

'Ow! Shit!' yelled Jack suddenly.

'What's happened?' I shrieked.

'Bloody stray shot hit my arm!' she shouted. Buddy snorted and tossed his head around.

'Ow! Oh my God! I've been hit in the eye!' A hot bit of pellet seared the corner of my eye. My entire body became rigid with shock and that was enough for Poppy. She made a strange grunting sound, pricked her ears up and barged to the front of the line then she went into her crazily fast trot.

'Whoa! Slow down!' I yelled, to no avail. I could almost hear her saying, *Slow down? Are you mad?*

By now the bridle path had joined an open field where it continued along the edge as a wide sandy path. Poppy broke into a canter and my foot slipped out of my left stirrup.

'Whoa!' I called out, fruitlessly. I felt completely unbalanced and full of panic at the thought of falling off. Behind me, all the other horses began to canter, which stressed Poppy out and sent her into a gallop.

'Oh my God!' I yelled as my right foot came out of the stirrup. I sat deep into the saddle and gripped tightly to the reins as my heart burst into a flurry of ectopic beats, triggering severe nausea. Behind me I could hear various yells and expletives and then, surprisingly, some peals of laughter from Gillian.

'Tally ho!' she hooted. Suddenly, memories of my childhood

experiences at the riding school pinged into the forefront of my mind. The joy of galloping fearlessly across country and how much I would have enjoyed this madness. The sudden change in my thoughts transferred to Poppy, who slowed instantly to a canter, which threw me onto her neck. Luckily, this slowed her right down to a trot and then she couldn't be bothered to trot any more so she went back into walk while I pushed myself back into the saddle. Behind me, all the horses slowed down and puffed and panted back into a walk.

'I'm so sorry,' I said, shame faced. 'I forgot she only responds to the word "stop"!'

'Sorry for what?' asked Gillian. 'That was tremendous fun and great exercise for our clearly unfit horses. Look at them all sweating!'

'Bloody hell,' laughed Jack, mopping her brow. 'Buddy will need to lie down for a week after that. Galloping is not his strong point.'

'Oh! They've stopped,' said Sapna and we all became aware of the silence. 'Thank God for that.'

'Phew,' I agreed, as my heart rhythm returned to normal. 'That was so stressful.'

'Stressful?' laughed Gillian. 'Not at all! It was a tonic for the system. We all need a bit of fun in life, don't you think?'

'My younger self would definitely agree with that, but my adult self thinks the opposite.'

'Oh dear. It sounds like you need a drop of the Bach remedy, mimulus. That will ease your worries and help you to enjoy the ride a bit more,' Gillian nodded knowingly.

Out of the corner of my eye I could see Jack raising her

eyebrows but fortunately she managed to control herself and said nothing. The rest of the ride passed without incident and we got to see the most stunning views of parkland in the distance, which belonged to the Deerwood Estate.

'That's a great place to ride,' said Sapna. 'We can go there next week if you like?'

'Marvellous idea,' agreed Gillian enthusiastically. 'We can take a picnic!'

'Sounds good to me,' nodded Jack.

When we reached the lane, we all went our separate ways just as the shotguns started up again in the distance. Poppy and Buddy completely ignored it as they were obviously too tired to care. But it reminded me of my eye, which suddenly began to sting.

'It's very red,' noted Jack after we had dismounted. 'Another millimetre to the left and that would have been a hospital visit.'

'Twats!' I muttered, inspecting it in my car's wing mirror.

Driving home, despite my eye, I managed to see the positive side of the horrible experience. It struck me how sensitive horses were. Just the simple act of Gillian laughing about it had made me feel relaxed and brave again. And this change within me had filtered through to Poppy, who instantly relaxed too. It was fascinating to observe how strongly my thoughts had the power to make her react for good or bad. But it was one thing being able to do it with someone else who is relaxed. How would I do it by myself? I wondered.

Chapter 12

The weekend came and went as fast as lightning but Monday morning presented me with a few hours of time. Usually, I would have filled that perfectly easily with various dull and mundane household chores but I decided I had to put my brave pants on and go for my first solo ride. Jack would not always be able to ride out with me so I had no choice, even though I was extremely nervous about it. The previous day I had watched with wonder at Florence during her riding lesson. Think Like a Pony was a truly inspiring place and it had given me much food for thought so I planned to try some of it out. A lot of it was very similar to the things I had learned in Wales.

What if those lunatic men are there, shooting again? I felt sick at the thought of it.

I wish we hadn't done this. Why have I moved to a field where there's no one to ride with?

The drive to the field should have been exciting and lovely to think that I would be there alone and not have to dodge the likes of Bitchy Louise or Bossy Morag. But instead, I was tense the entire journey. My arms were as stiff as a board and the pain in my shoulders shrieked of fear. It wasn't just the thought of the idiot men with shotguns. It was the whole responsibility of it all, especially the land management side of it. The field had been neglected for years and I had noticed a few rosettes of ragwort beginning to appear. Things like this had been taken care of at the previous yards but at this place it was down to us and I had zero knowledge of how to deal with poisonous plants. I pulled into the layby opposite the field and took a few deep breaths before going over to open the gate. Just as I put my hand out to unlock the padlock, I heard a loud rumble and crashing sound just round the bend in the lane.

'What the hell was that?' I wondered out loud and froze for a few moments before running to see what had happened.

'The bloody wall has collapsed!' I shouted, hardly able to believe my eyes. 'Oh my God! What am I supposed to do about this?'

I stood, open mouthed and dumbstruck, but then I realised that I had to move all the stones off the road quickly before someone had an accident. They weighed a ton. It was extremely annoying and time consuming but there was no other choice. I had to do it. I piled them up in front of what was left of that bit of wall, then my heart sank further when it dawned on me that I would have to tell Roger about it. I sent him a text because I didn't want to talk to him.

Oh shit! The horses could get out! My mind alerted me. I dashed into the field to see how big the gap in the wall was.

Oh thank God for that! In front of that section of wall was a line of stock fencing so the horses were safe. I took a deep breath and calmed myself down and was surprised to see Poppy standing nearby as if waiting for me.

'Oh hello,' I greeted as I remembered what my original plan had been. 'It's now or never to go out alone.' Poppy nodded her head as if in agreement. Obviously, it was probably a fly in her eye but to me it looked like she was saying yes. I felt that if I didn't get on and do it now, I would always find an excuse to not do it.

Oh hell. Is this safe? Memories of the shooting men popped into my head. But luckily all was quiet.

Is life ever safe? replied the wise part of my brain.

No, I suppose it isn't, I conceded.

Just get on with it and you can always get off if you need to. That realisation helped to calm me down and I stopped and took yet another deep breath.

Poppy looked at me quizzically. I rolled my shoulders and did my best to loosen the tension from my arms. Then I stepped forwards next to Poppy's shoulder and reached out to touch her. She took a deep breath and slightly lowered her head.

That's a good start, I said to myself as I put her headcollar on. I opened up my body to encourage her to take a step forward and we walked into the centre of the field together. I decided to do a bit of lunging first to 'get the tickle out of her toes', as my riding instructor, Elise, would say. So just to burn off any excess energy she may have we did walk, trot and canter. Then I decided I wanted to build up a deeper sense of connection, the way Florence had done with the riding school pony. It seemed like a sensible thing to do before riding out somewhere new so we went for a walk together round the entire field. All the while I had to fight myself to stop remembering the terrible hail of shotgun pellets.

If it's a regular thing round here, we're just going to have to get used to it, I kept telling myself.

But why should I get used to that? If it happens again, I'm calling the police. It's totally out of order!

Ok, call the police, but in the meantime it's not happening now so calm down.

Look at that bloody ragwort! It's everywhere! What the hell am I going to do about it?

The spiral of thoughts finally fizzled away as we approached the return up the field towards the shelter. A red kite came in to land ahead of us, which completely took my mind off worries. It was such an enormous bird. I stopped in awe to admire its beauty. The sun glinted on the golden colours of its feathers while it strutted about, as if showing off to me.

Wow! Just wow! How many people get to see a red kite walking around this close?

I suddenly heard a loud whirring noise that reverberated through my heart. Surprised, I looked up to see a pair of giant white geese flying overhead. The sound was so magnificent and wild that it made me cry. I watched them as they continued their flight over the top of the pine woods at the bottom edge of our back field and on towards the reservoir. I wiped my eyes and felt full of gratitude to have been able to witness the magic of nature so close. Just then, a large bold rabbit hopped past quite leisurely as if it didn't care about me or the red kite. I then remembered that red kites aren't hunting birds, they're scavengers who only eat things that are already dead. I smiled and felt deeply relaxed and ready to attempt the solo ride.

Jack had created two grooming stations inside the shelter, which I was looking forward to using. It felt extremely pleasant to have total peace and quiet, the only sounds were the distant hum of a tractor and the little birds tweeting in the hedge. I noticed that Poppy was more relaxed than she used to be while grooming, which was great. I tacked up, took a deep breath and led her into the carpark. Buddy didn't bother to raise his head from grazing which helped to keep Poppy calm.

Am I really doing this? Is it wise? Should I just ride in the field? Panic suddenly set in.

I walked my horses for miles before riding them, I suddenly remembered Jim's wise words. *Yes! I should walk her.*

I left her saddle on, clipped the lead rein to her bridle and felt much calmer about going out alone. I had no idea where I was going so I decided to keep it simple and do a very short circular route through the little village and back. Poppy walked out very calmly. It was not how I had expected her to be but I felt so relieved that I was able to relax my arms and look around and enjoy seeing the pretty, chocolate box cottages and beautiful woods.

'Hello! Can you help?' called a voice suddenly, jolting me out of my reverie. I looked around. On a wide muddy track, lower down a grassy bank, there was a woman on a small chestnut horse. 'He won't budge!' she shouted up to me.

'Oh dear,' I replied. 'I'll come to you!' I urged Poppy into a trot and I jogged along the lane until there was a clear way of getting down onto the track below.

'Come on, you bugger,' pleaded the lady. The horse began to walk backwards. 'No! Not that way!' she yelled. Poppy whinnied and the horse stopped, turned round and marched towards us with his ears pricked.

'Oh thank God for that! I was about to get off.' The lady grinned. She looked a similar age to me and had long red hair in a ponytail poking out from the back of her hat.

'Hello!' I grinned back. 'I'm Grace and this is Poppy.'

'I'm Wendy and this is Bastard.' She smirked.

'That's hilarious!'

'He's really called Denwyn but he's such a bloody bastard I don't know what to do.'

'Have you had him long?' I asked.

'No, he arrived two months ago. And he's fine leading out in hand like you're doing but as soon as I get on it's a different story. We've literally only come from there.' Wendy pointed towards a barn.

'Oh! Is that a livery yard?'

'No, it's my in-laws' farm. They don't like horses so the whole thing is turning out to be a bit of a nightmare. But I've always wanted a horse and I got offered this one for free. Now I know why he was free.'

'How can anyone not like horses?' I was stunned.

'I know. It's so weird,' laughed Wendy. 'But they don't like him and the more he plays up the more they complain about him. So, I need to show them he's a good horse.'

'Do you think he might settle a bit more if he follows us?' I asked. 'Maybe I'll ride now if I can find somewhere to climb on. She's too tall for me to get on from the ground.'

'Oh, that would be great. There's a bit of old wall just there you could use. Are you sure you don't mind us tagging along?'

'No, it would be lovely. I'm new here so I have no idea where to ride,' I replied as I tentatively climbed onto the wall and mounted. I was very relieved to have met someone to ride with.

'It's really nice in Deerwood, shall we go there?' suggested Wendy.

'I'm happy to go anywhere.' I nodded.

Wendy told me which way to go so I turned Poppy round and urged her to walk on. She was having none of it. Instead, she lifted her tail and shot a powerful jet of wee all over Denwyn. Unfortunately, it hit Wendy's legs too.

'Oh my God I am so sorry!' I was mortified. Wendy threw her head back and guffawed.

'That's hilarious! It stinks,' she laughed, tears streaming down her face.

Poppy decided to play up to her amused audience and once again jetted out a stream of pungent wee.

'Poppy stop it,' I pleaded.

'Good heavens!' exclaimed a rather sharp voice. I looked round to see a most stern-looking old lady walking past with a Golden Retriever trotting by her side.

'Your horse has just voided her bladder on my dog,' said the not-too-pleased lady.

'I'm so sorry!' I was extremely embarrassed.

'I don't know why people have horses. They're more trouble than they're worth,' she replied, heatedly.

'Hi Margaret, this is my new friend Grace. Grace, this is my mother-in-law,' said Wendy raising her eyebrows. As you can imagine, I was lost for words. Margaret said a curt hello.

'I suppose I'll go and wash my dog in the stream now,' she said as she marched off.

'Oh hell,' I said after she had disappeared into the woods. 'I am so sorry.'

But Wendy just laughed. 'It's fine. She can't stand me or Denwyn. Let's get out of here quick!'

Eventually, I managed to persuade Poppy to get a move on and we hurried off towards the bridle path that would take us into Deerwood. It was a beautiful path lined with hedges of holly and here and there an overgrown rose bush coming back to life. All the while, Wendy chattered about her despair with Denwyn and how he hadn't turned out to be the horse she always dreamed of having. He was very jumpy and nervy.

'You're so lucky to have such a chilled-out horse,' sighed Wendy.

'Er, yes,' I replied, with mild amusement. 'She's not always like this. She can be extremely stressy and moody sometimes. It's been a lot of hard work to be honest.'

'Wow really? I can't imagine that seeing how relaxed she is now,' said Wendy as Denwyn decided to jump sideways into the hedge for no apparent reason. 'Bloody hell, Denwyn! It was just a robin.' I was very relieved that Poppy was able to ignore Denwyn's behaviour and keep walking in a relaxed way. It was surprising to say the least.

After a while, the path wound its way into a rhododendron walk and presently we came to a beautifully planted track which had a sign saying 'Private No Entry!' It was a shame because it looked so inviting. There were enormous green, leafy plants that looked like something from a rainforest and a wide stream flowed down the edge of the path. The water was so clear and inviting.

'Shall we go down here?' Wendy suggested. 'It looks so much nicer than the public path.' We both looked around and saw no one.

'Yes let's.' I grinned and we almost tiptoed onto the forbidden footpath.

It was lined on one side with Scotch pine trees so the smell was quite intoxicating, and underfoot the surface was beautifully soft.

'It's a perfect canter track,' I said.

'Oi!' shouted a man stepping out from behind a tree. 'This is private! Can't you read?' He looked us up and down scowling. 'You shouldn't be on here. You horse riders are so up yourselves. You think you can ride anywhere! Well you can't ride here!'

'I'd like to see you try and stop us, you miserable sod,' replied Wendy and she urged Denwyn into a canter. Poppy quickly followed and we shot off down the path with the man shouting after us.

'Oh my God,' I laughed as we careered round a corner, up a hill and into the depths of the woods. 'Where the hell are we?'

'No idea!' shouted Wendy as she pulled Denwyn back into a trot and then a walk. 'Well he can canter and he can stop. That's good to know!' We mopped our brows and had a look around.

'I don't know where that bit of rebellion came from,' Wendy apologised. 'I'm not usually like that but he was so rude!'

'He was horrible. We can't go back now he's probably waiting for us with a shotgun.'

'Yes! Oh heck. Let's head that way and it should lead us back to Acer, fingers crossed.'

Riding through the woods made me feel like I was ten years old and back at the riding school on a treasure hunt. If I had known then that one day my dream of owning a horse would come true, I would have burst with joy.

'Oh bugger,' said Wendy suddenly. We had come to a gate which bizarrely was hanging open.

'What is it?' I asked, suddenly feeling less like a ten-year-old girl and more like a grown woman trespassing on private land who should know better.

'It looks like we're about to walk into the Birkdale Farm set,' Wendy grimaced. 'But there's no other way if we don't want to go back the way we came.'

'Birkdale Farm?' I repeated in surprise.

'Yes, you know? The soap opera? They film it here,' replied

Wendy. 'Bloody hope they aren't filming right now. And I really hope their security guards aren't around. They're ex-Gurkhas apparently.'

'Oh no. That sounds a bit disturbing. What should we do?'

'I think we have to just wing it,' Wendy laughed nervously and asked Denwyn to walk on. 'Come on! Walk on!' Denwyn refused to move. 'Could you go in front? Hopefully he'll follow you.'

'Come on, Poppy,' I asked nervously. Poppy wouldn't budge. 'Oh come on now! Walk on!'

'Walk on, Denwyn Wendy flapped her legs and urged him on to no avail.

'Poppy will you just get going?' I squeezed my legs firmly and jiggled around in the saddle as if that might help. It made no difference at all.

'Denwyn! Will you bloody walk on?' Denwyn walked backwards into Poppy.

'Poppy! You are driving me mad. Come on now!' Poppy walked sideways and bashed my leg on a tree. 'Ow! For God's sake, Poppy.' I was furious. Suddenly, she decided it was ok and walked forwards onto the set of the Birkdale Farm Village. Denwyn promptly followed.

'Oh shit they're filming over there!' squeaked Wendy as she pointed over towards a camera crew outside one of the houses.

'Oh hell,' I replied nervously. 'Isn't this just a village? Can't we just say we live here?'

'No,' Wendy shook her head. 'It's a fake village! Looks real though doesn't it?'

'Are you kidding? This is fake? It looks so real!' I looked around at the houses. It all looked believable to me.

'Oh bollocks. They've seen us! What do we do?' hissed Wendy as the crew looked over at us.

'Keep going,' I said. 'Don't look at them. Let's just ride as if we do actually live here.'

'Ok!'

We rode nonchalantly down the very realistic fake lane until we were very close to the film crew.

'Cut!' yelled one of them. The entire crew stared at us.

'Can I ask what you're doing here, ladies?' a man who was possibly the director looked at us quizzically.

'We're extras,' I replied without thinking. 'We're the village horse riders.'

'Oh, right. I didn't know we were having riders today. Phil did you order any riders?' The man leafed through the script and scratched his head. 'It doesn't mention horses here. Who arranged the riders?'

A young lad appeared from behind a large camera. 'I don't think I did? Could it have been Zainab?'

'Sorry ladies, there seems to have been a bit of a mix-up again. We really don't need horses in this particular scene but if you head back towards the carpark, please do help yourself to some lunch and obviously you will still get paid for your time,' said the man apologetically.

'Oh that's a shame. Never mind.' Wendy smiled politely and thank goodness both horses walked sensibly towards the gate that led out to the carpark.

'Wow!' we both exploded with laughter when we were safely out of earshot. 'Crikey! How lucky was that?'

'I thought we were going to be in serious trouble,' gasped Wendy. 'Let's get back home before we get arrested!'

The ride back through the farm and bridleways was, fortunately, without any more incidents and Denwyn walked well.

'He's knows he's going home now,' said Wendy as we trotted down the road towards her in-laws' farm yard.

'Well that was a ride to remember,' I laughed and we arranged to meet again.

I rode the rest of the way back to the field alone, grinning crazily about all that had just happened and once again enjoyed the sound of the birds and the sounds of the distant farm machinery. Buddy was still grazing without a care in the world and although the dreaded ragwort popped back into my mind, I felt a deep sense of peace, which was the opposite of what I had expected for my first ride out without Jack. I untacked Poppy, gave her a kiss and turned her loose.

'You'll have to pay for that bloody wall!' shouted a familiar voice. A very red-faced Roger stormed into the carpark.

'Pardon?' I was rendered stunned by his peculiar silk, paisley shawl flapping around his neck. It looked odd next to his tweed shooting jacket and perfectly ironed jeans.

'The fecking wall! Your bloody nuisance horses have obviously pushed it down!' he waved his arm around gesturing at the big gap in the stone wall, his face twisted up with anger. My heartrate increased twenty-fold.

'No they didn't!' I replied.

'Of course they did!' spluttered Roger, pulling his shawl off with rage. 'They're always scratching their big backsides on it!' He marched past me to inspect the damage. I followed him in a haze of stress.

What the hell? I'm not paying for his wall!

'There's a wire fence in front of it,' I rallied triumphantly. 'They couldn't possibly have pushed it over!'

'Hmmm. Phht,' snarled Roger, clearly disappointed. 'They probably pushed their bottoms under it and pushed the wall over.'

'How could they do that?' I couldn't believe my ears. 'They'd cut themselves!'

'Well, I suppose I'll have to pay for it this time but don't bloody do it again. I'm not made of money!' He waved his shawl at me and strode away with his head held high and his ginger ponytail bobbing up and down.

I stumbled back into the carpark and sat down, my mind reeling.

Christ almighty, what a terrifying man! I had to take several deep breaths before I felt calm enough to text Jack and tell her all about it.

'Bloody nutter!' she replied. 'He's worse than Valerie.'

Why have we come here? This is just too stressful. I drove home feeling so uptight that the thought of housework was actually a welcome distraction.

Chapter 13

'Don't go mad but I've done something!' texted Jack just as I was coming round from a terrible night of stressful dreams about Roger and ragwort. I had actually laid awake for hours worrying about it all. I re-read the text and took a deep breath dreading the worst. I was late and I had to hurry up and make breakfasts for all of us and a packed lunch for Florence. My heart missed several beats as I typed my reply.

'What have you done?' Jack had a history of doing insane things on the spur of the moment.

'I've bought a pony!'

'What? Oh no!' I said out loud just as my phone started ringing.

'Jack what the hell have you done?' I laughed nervously.

'It's my dad's fault!' she blurted. 'Well ok it was my idea first, but he encouraged me to actually go ahead and do it.'

'Oh blimey, you nutter. I'm just making breakfast so I'm putting you on speaker and Florence is in the kitchen, so try not to swear.'

'Well my dad wanted to go to the livestock auction yesterday and there were some ponies for sale. So I said I thought it might be a good idea to buy a pony and sell it on to make a bit of money at the field.'

'Right?' I took a deep breath to calm myself down. Florence was listening in to our conversation, her face alight with excitement.

'I figured your Florence could ride it and then we could get some good videos and get a good price for it. So my dad started bidding on this pony and nobody else bid so we had to buy him. Are you cross?'

'Yay! Daddy! Aunty Jack has bought me a pony!' shrieked Florence as James walked into the kitchen.

'She's done what?' James looked shell shocked.

'Oh hi James!' shouted d Jack. 'I've bought a pony! But don't worry it's to sell on!'

'Oh thank God for that,' replied James. 'Right, I've got to dash, see you later.' James gave me and Florence a kiss, grabbed his breakfast and hurried off to work.

'Has he gone?' asked Jack.

'Yes, why?' I asked.

'Well er I don't know how to tell you this next bit.'

'Oh God. Do I need to sit down?' I could feel my blood pressure rising.

'Don't be mad but, well, oh heck.'

'Just say it before I have a heart attack!'

'Ok. I bought a three-year-old too ...'

'Yayyyyy!' shrieked Florence and she began dancing around the kitchen. This set Wrexford off and the pair of them jumped around clearly having a tremendous time.

'A three-year-old?' I sat down on the nearest chair which turned out to be the dog's crate. It almost collapsed under me.

'It was just a spur of the moment decision. She's really cute! I promise you will absolutely love her.' I could almost hear Jack grimacing.

'Right,' was all I could say. 'I'll come up as soon as I've dropped Florence at school.'

'Ok see you soon!'

The drive to the field was riddled with anxiety. Half of my brain was chuntering on about *ragwort and what are we going to do about it?* and the other half was in free-fall panic mode about *how the hell are we going to cope with a three-year-old horse?* Between the two subjects my mind was at bursting point. I skidded to a halt in the layby opposite the field and I almost fell out of my car in the scramble to get to the gate.

'Oh God,' I gasped as I beheld the sight of broken fencing and a young ginger and white skewbald pony running round and round in the carpark. 'What the hell has happened?'

'Shit the bed!' called Jack, who was trying to catch the youngster but with no luck. 'She's absolutely trashed everything. Look at the shelter! No don't look at the shelter I'll fix it I promise!' I looked over at the shelter where part of one side was hanging limply as if an elephant had reversed into it.

'How can one small animal do so much damage?' I couldn't believe my eyes.

'Oh my God.' My gaze suddenly fell on the other new pony, a very pretty 13.2hh grey Welsh section C. 'What's he doing?'

'Oh heck! Maverick stop it!' Jack leaped over the crumpled fence and dashed over to the pony, who was attempting to mount Poppy. For a small chap his penis was remarkably large and he looked like he meant business despite the fact he was not actually capable of mounting Poppy due to her being more than twice his size. Credit to him though he wasn't letting that tiny detail put him off trying. Jack flailed her arms around and eventually Poppy kicked out at him and trotted away with the lovestruck lothario in hot pursuit. All that was missing was the theme tune from Benny Hill as they circled round and round the top half of the front field.

'I suppose it's giving her a bit of exercise,' I muttered.

'I'm so sorry! What have I done?' Jack looked distraught.

'Now then! What's going on here?' We looked round to find Jack's dad grinning at the mayhem. He leaped over the carpark gate and expertly grabbed the young pony. 'Pass me a head collar!'

'The guy said she's never had one on,' replied Jack. 'I wanted to get her used to it gently like what it says in the foal training book!'

'Never mind books! She's not a foal any more neither. Pass me a head collar! She'll get used to it now!'

Jack grabbed a small head collar that she had bought for her and threw it to her dad. In one swift move he had it on her head and told her in no uncertain terms that she had to stand still. She clearly understood him because she stood stock-still. Probably feeling secure that someone with knowledge had taken charge.

'Right, Grace love,' he said. 'You get in here and hold this 'un while I go and sort out Mr Loverman over there.' I climbed over the gate and held tight onto the young pony, who by now was very tired and was almost nodding off to sleep.

'Right, you bugger!' said Jack's dad. 'You can put your thingy away for a start!' Headcollar and lead rope in hand, he marched over to Maverick, who was still trotting round and round after Poppy, who was not amused at all. He threw the lead rope in such a way that it wound round Maverick's neck, which startled him and fortunately stopped him in his tracks. He allowed the head collar to be put on him and he was marched over to the carpark.

'We're gonna have to make him a separate paddock. Looks like he's a rig,' said Jack's dad, nodding knowledgably.

'What's a rig?' I asked, wide-eyed.

'It's where its nuts are in its belly so he's not been castrated. Either that or he was used as a stud and castrated later, so he'll still behave like a stallion.'

'I didn't know you knew so much about horses, Dad,' said Jack in surprise.

'I know a lot about beasts,' laughed her dad. 'Right let's get this mess sorted out.'

Jack and I held onto the errant ponies while her dad fixed the broken carpark fencing, whistling merrily all the while. He then hopped over the fence into the field and swiftly sorted out the shelter in what appeared to be five seconds flat.

'That's that sorted,' he said, looking pleased with himself. 'Now we'd best get a paddock sorted out for that little sod.' He looked around and decided the best place to do it was the top bit of the front field. 'Hang on a moment.' He wandered off to his car and came back with a few roles of electric sheep netting and a battery. 'This'll do the job.' In no time at all he had erected a paddock in which Maverick could not get to Poppy.

'Right! I'd best get the dog walked now. See you both later.' He waved cheerily and went on his way.

'Thank God for your dad,' I sighed as he drove away.

'Yeah he can be helpful sometimes,' nodded Jack. 'Oh shit, Grace, what have I done?'

'What you always do,' I laughed. 'I think we need to think about getting a new owner for Maverick as soon as possible.'

'God yes. But how?' Jack seemed tired from the whole shenanigan and she sat down on the mounting block. The younger pony had settled down to sleep at my feet. She was a cute little traditional Gypsy Cob with lots of thick mane and feather. 'She's called Toffee,' said Jack, nodding at her.

'That's a great name,' I said. 'Florence will probably love her.'

'I can't believe she broke the fence,' said Jack. 'Oh no, what's he doing?'

Maverick was not happy in his new paddock and he was trotting round and round, neighing. Buddy wandered over to see him, which settled him down a bit, but Poppy completely ignored him, glad that he was away from her.

'I'll bring Florence up after school and we can crack on with making videos so that you can sell him on,' I suggested.

'Good plan,' agreed Jack, jumping to her feet. 'I'll set up a school area next to the shelter, then we'll look a bit more professional.'

'That's a great idea but I've got to go to work now so I can't help.'

'Good,' laughed Jack. 'I know what you're like with DIY!'

I grinned and set off back to the car to get to work.

What a nightmare! My brain launched into stress mode.

How will we cope with a young pony that trashes everything and a pony that's clearly a stallion? I felt sick with the responsibility of it. *And the bloody ragwort too. What the hell to do about that?*

By the time I arrived home I was mentally exhausted, which wasn't such a bad thing because it meant my brain stopped talking at me. I prepared my therapy room and had a quick snack just in time to open the door to my first client.

'Now do tell me what's the latest at the field?' trilled Lady Alexa as she almost bounced up the stairs to my therapy room. 'I've been so looking forward to hearing all about it! I do think you are very brave to be the mistress of your own land. I'd never dare take on such a huge undertaking.'

'Brave or stupid?' I laughed. 'You won't believe what Jack's just done.' I poured out the whole sorry tale.

'Oh dear,' laughed Alexa. 'It sounds like Jack's dad is a useful chap to have on hand though, even if he did do a silly thing, bidding on the pony.'

'Yes, he's great with farm animals, thank goodness. But I have no idea how we're going to cope with this extra stress.'

'I have to admit, having dealt with many young horses, you are correct. It is a massively stressful thing to take on, especially when you've never done it before. But if you need me to come and help then I will pop over!'

'Oh wow! Thank you so much.' I was so relieved to hear that. 'It's the ragwort that's doing my head in the most. I have no idea what to do about it and every day there's more of it.'

'Oh heck! Land management is not my forte. You'll have to Google it.'

'Oh yes, of course! That's a good idea. I don't know why I haven't done that already, I'm an idiot.' I breathed a sigh of relief.

The afternoon disappeared rapidly and suddenly it was school pickup time. As usual, the bitchy mums were standing in their coven-like group talking about complete rubbish. I looked at them and momentarily envied their seemingly stress-free lives.

What have you airheads got to think about? I wondered. *Should I have a manicure or a pedicure? Oh dear I've run out of mascara!*

I was so annoyed by them.

You don't have to think about ragwort or mad ponies running riot!

Fortunately, Florence came skipping out of school before I could wind myself up any further and then my mind settled as I realised it must be very boring to be them.

'Can we go and see the new ponies?' asked Florence, jumping up and down. 'Please! Please! Please!'

'Yes, I've brought your riding clothes. Why don't you run back inside and get changed in the toilets?' I handed Florence the bag of clothes and she dashed back into school. In no time at all she ran back out, showing off to her school friends about going to see *her new ponies*. One particular girl, who was the unfortunate daughter of a bitchy mum, looked really hopeful and asked her mother if she could have a pony.

'Ooh no!' replied the mother, her face twisting up in utter disgust at the mere thought of it. 'They're very dirty animals!' The little girl's face fell and she looked over at Florence with a tinge of envy. I felt so sorry for her to have such an unpleasant mother. It made me feel like I was quite a fantastic mum, for a change.

'Ok, let's get going. Jack's waiting for us with her camera,' I said to Florence, who let out a whoop of joy and sped to the car at top speed.

All the way to the field, Florence was singing songs from Andrew Lloyd Webber musicals to express her tremendous excitement. I, on the other hand, had a terrible running commentary running through my mind.

What are we going to do if nobody wants to buy Maverick?

What the hell are we going to do with Toffee?

Florence will want to keep her, and I have no idea how to train a horse from scratch and neither does Jack, and we can't afford another horse.

And what the hell am I going to do about the ragwort? How much will all that cost?

With a deep sigh, I pulled into the layby and opened the gate into the field.

'Stop it, you big turd!' shouted Jack as she ran over to Maverick. He had clearly managed to escape the confines of his separation paddock and was busy humping Toffee, who didn't seem too bothered about it.

'Mummy, what are the ponies doing?' Florence asked with the innocence of childhood. I had no idea how to respond.

'Oh, er, I'm not sure. It must be a game?'

'What's that big stick on his tummy, Mummy?' she asked quizzically.

'Ah well erm.' I was lost for words.

'Is that his willy, Mummy?'

'How do you know about willies?' I was shocked.

'Wrexford has a willy, Mummy! Everyone knows about willies,' Florence laughed her head off.

Jack managed to catch Maverick and detach him from Toffee. She led him over to us and Florence threw her arms around his neck and gave him a kiss.

'Can I ride him?' she asked, almost bursting with excitement.

'Let's see what he's like when we give him a brush first eh?' Jack grinned. 'We need to make sure he's ok.' Florence nodded.

'At Think Like a Pony we check the ponies are feeling good before we ride,' she said. 'Shall I show you what we do?'

'Yes please!' said Jack and I simultaneously.

It was fascinating to watch Florence take a deep breath and shake the tension out of her shoulders. Once she felt sufficiently loose, she put her hand on Maverick's shoulder. Maverick was very relaxed and appeared to be interested in Florence.

'Good boy,' she said and then began to brush him. 'Now we have to walk him around so that we get a connection.'

'Right,' said Jack, nodding earnestly. 'Here you are then.' She passed the lead rope to Florence and we all walked around the top of the field together. I didn't dare let her do it alone in case Maverick turned out to be dangerous. Fortunately, he was very chilled out and walked nicely. He had obviously been very well schooled and he seemed very happy to have the attention.

'Ok, Aunty Jack. He's ready for his saddle and bridle now.' Florence was very excited as Jack went to her van and revealed the small saddle and bridle she had bought at the auction. They were a good fit, which was lucky.

'I've made a school so you can ride him in there,' said Jack leading us over to the shelter, next to which was a very large, separate rectangle of grass which had been fenced off with wooden posts and blue rope. It was actually very impressive, but Jack dismissed it as just a basic thing. 'Even you could make this, Grace,' she laughed.

'I don't think so,' I replied. It felt very exciting to have a proper schooling area and I couldn't wait to go in there with Poppy.

'Right let's get you on,' said Jack, giving Florence a leg-up. I held my breath anxiously in case Maverick reared or bucked but thank goodness he did neither. He walked and trotted very nicely and even managed to go over a large branch which Jack had cut down to see how he would cope with obstacles.

'Excellent,' I said. 'He seems like a great little pony.'

'He is in here,' agreed Jack. 'But what on earth are we going to do about his behaviour out there? That electric sheep netting didn't keep him in.'

'Can we take him home?' asked Florence. 'He can live in our garden!'

'No we can't take him home.'

'Tonight he'll have to stay in the carpark while I think what to do,' sighed Jack. 'Let's go and see Toffee.'

'Yay!' squealed Florence and as I untacked Maverick, they went over to see Toffee, who was standing on top of the muck heap kicking poo into the field. Florence thought it was hilarious as Jack waved her arms around furiously trying to stop her making such a mess.

The drive home was peppered with repetitive questions from Florence, namely, 'Can we keep Maverick?' and 'Can we keep Toffee?' It was very wearing to have to repeat 'No' over and over again. I wanted to be able to say 'Yes!' because I remembered how badly I had wanted a pony when I was her age. But the reality of having a pony meant more expense and the inevitable moment when the child grows out of the pony, and then what do you do? I personally couldn't sell a pony just because it was too small, but then what happens? You end up with at least three different ponies of various heights and that would just be an impossible expense. James would have heart failure at the thought of it. So I had to remind her that one day she would be tall enough to ride Poppy and that made her happy.

Chapter 14

I dashed up to the field as soon as I could to see what, if anything, had happened overnight with the two new hooligans. Fortunately, Maverick was still in the carpark but Toffee was nowhere to be seen. I went to find her thinking she was probably playing in the stream or something.

'Oh my God,' I gasped as my blood turned to ice. My heart began beating so fast I thought I would faint. 'Shitting hell!'

I grabbed my phone to call Jack. 'Pick up for God's sake!' I tried to call again but still she didn't answer. 'Oh God what do I do? What do I do?' I was not equipped to deal with a pony who was stuck in such a way.

'How did you get your front legs over the barbed wire?' I couldn't see how she had managed to do it without cutting herself to ribbons. 'Don't move, Toffee! Just keep still!' This last request was, fortunately, completely unnecessary because she was standing very still as if she understood the danger she was in, but I was completely frozen. I had no idea what to do. Suddenly I became aware that a tractor had come to a halt on the lane opposite to where I was standing.

'Oh dear! Looks like someone's been a bit daft,' said the driver. I looked up to see an oldish-looking, wiry man peering down at us. 'I thought she looked a bit odd when I came past earlier. Do you need a hand?'

'Yes please!' I was so relieved. The old man leaped out of the cab and sprang over the wall like a gymnast and had a look at the situation.

'Aye, right. You'll need some wire cutters for that.' He nodded knowingly. The man stank to high heaven of cow shit, which wasn't surprising as his grey overalls were splattered in the stuff.

'I haven't got any wire cutters!' I wailed. I was terrified that Toffee would suddenly start to panic and end up slicing her tummy open.

'No bother, I've got some here.' The man pulled a pair of wire cutters out of his pocket. 'I'm always having to cut me own beasts free.' He clipped the top strand of barbed wire and then the short, skinny man lifted Toffee back over the stock fence as if she was as light as a feather. She snorted a sort of thank you and casually mooched off as if nothing major had just happened. I was amazed. If that had been Poppy she would have gone berserk and eviscerated herself.

'Don't they need ear tags?' asked the old man, cocking his head to one side.

'Ear tags?' I repeated.

'You know? The big yeller things like what cows and sheep have to wear?'

'Ah yes. No they don't.'

'Oh right,' he nodded, scratching his wispy grey hair. 'That's peculiar isn't it? So do they not get eaten eventually like?'

'Eaten?' I was horrified. 'No! They're pets!'

'Oh. Right.' The old man nodded and scratched his head again. 'I've never understood why people have horses. Spendin' a lot o' brass for nowt I reckon. But it teks all sorts to mek a world doesn't it?'

'Er yes, I suppose it does.'

'I'm Adam by the way. I own the farm over there.' He pointed over to where Wendy kept her horse, Denwyn.

'Oh are you Wendy's father-in-law?' I was fascinated to meet him.

'Aye I am. Well cheerio!' and before I could say anything else he leaped back over the wall and into his tractor. He gave a little wave as he drove off. I watched him drive away feeling slightly stunned by the abrupt end to the conversation when suddenly a large black sack, followed by a load of wood, came flying over the wall next to me.

'Watch out!' shouted Jack as she hurled a few more bits of wood into the field. 'Give us a hand with this!' Jack pulled a bath out of the back of her van and lifted it over the wall for me to pull into the field.

'What's all this for?' I asked, but she'd got back in her van and was driving up the lane to the field gate. Presently, she trotted over to me brandishing several tools.

'I'm making a horse,' she panted.

'A horse?' I replied.

'Yes. A wooden horse to keep Maverick company when he's in his paddock. He can't live in the carpark forever.'

'Right,' I nodded. 'Can today get any more weird?'

'Why what else has happened?' asked Jack.

'Toffee was stuck half way over the barbed wire near that wall and then I met the local farmer, who cut her free and then he walked off midway through a conversation.'

'Oh how funny. But not funny about Toffee. What a nightmare is she ok? Has she cut herself?'

'No thank God.'

'Phew! What a stress.' She looked over at Toffee, who was busy chewing some of the fence. 'Glad that ended ok. Right, let me get on with this.'

It was fascinating to watch Jack sawing bits of wood and hammering nails in. She was such a talented woodworker. She made a frame and then attached four posts, turned it over and then we balanced the bath on top. Jack then laid underneath it and fiddled around with some metal things that I am ashamed to admit I have no idea what they were. However, it resulted in the whole contraption becoming very sturdy. Jack gave it a firm shake.

'That's good.' She nodded and then started working on some other pieces of wood, whistling a little tune. In front of my eyes, she created what looked like a horse's head made out of the pieces of wood.

'Wow! That's amazing!' I said, deeply impressed by her skill.

'Oh it's nothing.' She blushed modestly. 'Here, you hold it while I attach its hair.' She pulled a big bunch of horse hair out of her pocket. 'This is some of Buddy's tail. I cut it off last night when I got the idea to make this. He's got loads of hair so he didn't mind.' Jack created a forelock and then, using some glue, she stuck it on the head. Somehow or other she then attached the head to another length of wood and that became the neck. This whole section was then connected to the bath along with a 'tail' at the back end.

'The head looks brilliant,' I said. 'But I'm not sure he's going to be fooled by the rest of it.' I tapped the bath.

'Don't worry.' Jack grinned and rummaged around in the large sack. 'Now the finishing touch.' She pulled out a slightly muddy horse rug and put it on the wooden horse. It was perfect. The rug completely covered the bath and the wooden neck. 'Let's see if she works.'

'She?' I asked.

'Yes, she's called Valerie,' Jack guffawed with laughter.

'Brilliant idea!'

We carried Valerie up the field and stood back and watched. Maverick whinnied at it over the carpark fence and Buddy and Poppy trotted over, snorting and tossing their heads. They circled the fake horse a few times and then started to sniff it. Buddy gave it a bit of a kick but luckily it survived. In no time at all, the pair of them began grazing next to the wooden statue.

'How funny,' I chuckled.

'Great! Now let's get it into Maverick's pen and see what he does with it,' Jack said. We carried the horse into the separate area and then Jack went to get Maverick. Toffee trotted over to check it out too and she must have approved because she kept whinnying at it. Maverick trotted round and round the wooden horse and then he began to attempt to mount it.

'Oh my good God!' Jack's jaw dropped open. 'What's wrong with him?'

'He's a sex pest,' I sighed. 'I hope he doesn't break it.'

'Stop it, you dirty bugger!' Jack ran over to Maverick waving her arms about. It didn't put him off. He stopped in his own time, which was around ten minutes. Miraculously, Valerie survived the ordeal, which was very impressive considering she was made of wood and an old bath tub.

'Finally.' Jack nodded when Maverick settled down to graze. She flopped to the floor and fanned herself. 'What have I done?'

'What do you mean?' I asked.

'Why did I buy him and Toffee? I have no idea how to sell a pony and I have no idea how to train a horse. Oh God, what's she doing now?' Jack looked over at Toffee, who was pawing at the water trough.

'Well,' I replied, 'I think step one should be to work out how you want to sell Maverick.'

'Even though he's a pain in the arse I don't want to take him to the sales. He could end up in a terrible home. But how can I sell him to a young kid when he humps everything?'

'Hmmm, yes that might not go down too well, especially if he tries it while he's being ridden,' I conceded. 'Maybe you could aim the adverts at small adults?'

'Oh, good idea. Yes, we need a small adult. But it would have to be a really small adult for him! And where and how do I make these adverts?' It was unusual to see Jack unravel. Usually she was so confident and full of common sense.

'I can have a go at writing something if you like and then we can stick notices in all the horsey shops and livery yards, that would be a start. And then how about online? There must be websites specifically for selling horses?' I replied, feeling strange to be the practical one.

'Oh brilliant, thank you.' Jack seemed a bit happier and she jumped to her feet. 'What to do about this ragwort?' The sudden reminder of ragwort made me feel like a lead balloon. I sighed deeply.

'I can't stand the ragwort worry. It keeps me awake at night,' I admitted.

'I've been too busy worrying about Maverick and Toffee so it's only because of looking at it now that I remembered. It'll cost a fortune to spray all this land and why should we when it's not our field? That silly cow Anna has left it in a right mess here.'

'I wouldn't even know what to spray. And surely whatever kills ragwort can't be good for horses?'

'Shall we pull it?' asked Jack, heaving on a large plant. It wouldn't budge it was so deeply rooted. 'Yikes! That's not moving any time soon.'

'Don't touch that dreadful weed without gloves on!' shouted a familiar voice. We both jumped out of our skins and spun round to see Gillian. She was dressed as if for a garden party with royalty, in a dusky pink satin dress and cream jacket with a large sunhat. She made for an interesting sight but I suppose it was a sunny day and pleasantly warm for spring. She opened the gate and came over to us.

'I'm just getting my steps in and I knew exactly what you were up to as soon as I saw you. Oh dear you do have rather a lot of ragwort in here.' Gillian scanned the field with expert eyes.

'We have no idea what to do about it. Should we spray it or pull it?' I asked.

'Good God!' replied Gillian aghast. 'You should do neither! Pulling it will make it spread like billyo. Did you know that if you leave even a tiny bit of root that's enough to make ten more of the blasted things?'

'Really? No, I didn't know that,' I was stunned.

'Yes, it's a crafty little fellow is ragwort. And spraying it will just ruin your grazing unless you want only grass. I am of the opinion that a horse needs a broader diet and I also don't want any toxic chemicals in my animals.'

'So what should we do?' asked Jack.

'Homeopathy,' replied Gillian, nodding her head. 'Homeopathy every time!'

'Homey what?' asked Jack, perplexed.

'Homeopathy. It's where you use a very diluted amount of the disease, in this case ragwort, and you sprinkle it on the field, preferably during a full moon, and then you affirm that you don't want any more ragwort in the field. It worked well for me. I don't have any ragwort now.'

I could see Jack's expression so I swiftly intervened. 'That sounds interesting, Gillian. I'm not really sure how that would actually work though.'

'Never fear! Tonight is a full moon so I shall take a snippet of your ragwort and will prepare the remedy now. Let's meet at eight p.m. tonight and we shall give it a go!' There seemed to be no stopping Gillian and before Jack could open her mouth, she took a piece of ragwort and walked off.

'What just happened? Tell me we haven't just agreed to do the type of mad shit that Alex would do?' asked Jack when she finally felt able to speak.

'It seems that way, yes.' I shrugged.

'What the hell is homeopathy? Is it really a thing?' asked Jack, furiously trying to understand the concept.

'It is a thing yes and actually I used it on Florence when she was a baby and it worked really well,' I replied, remembering how certain remedies had completely cured her of colic and teething pains.

'What? You sprinkled a load of ragwort on her and it made her better? What the hell?'

I laughed my head off. 'No! Not ragwort! There are loads of different remedies for different ailments. You must have heard of arnica?'

'Oh yes. I used arnica cream on Buddy and that was really good. Is that homeopathy?'

'Yes, but not the sort of homeopathy Gillian is suggesting. I really don't think that it's going to get rid of ragwort from a field. That's just completely mad.'

'I wonder if she's got a remedy for him, he's at it again,' Jack pointed to Maverick, who had resumed his unhealthy interest in Valerie. 'What the hell is wrong with him? Stop it, Maverick!' she shouted. Maverick stopped and scratched his leg as if nothing had happened. 'Bloody weird pony.'

'So are we really going to come here tonight to do a crazy ritual?' I asked.

'Well, we can't not turn up can we?' Jack replied, pulling a face. 'And anything that's free is worth a go. Alex would love this. Don't tell her, for God's sake or we'll have her turning up too.' We both laughed and walked round the field to check how much of a problem the ragwort was.

'God it's bad, isn't it?' said Jack as we spotted more and more of the tell-tale rosettes popping up everywhere. It felt like they were laughing at us. The more we looked, the more we found and the tighter my chest became. I felt so guilty that I had put Poppy in a field full of poison. I wanted to cry but I choked it back and sighed instead.

'Well it can't harm to do Gillian's mad ritual can it?' I said.

'No,' Jack agreed. 'It's something to do tonight instead of watching tv.'

After a day of boring chores, I have to admit I was secretly looking forward to the evening's adventure. I leaped outside with excitement and got into the car. The sky was very clear, full of stars that I rarely bothered to notice and a great big, full moon. It was cold but a nice sort of cold that was sharp and dry, unlike the horrid wet cold that penetrates into your bones. The drive to the field felt very unusual in the dark. It was a different world with all the evening animals flitting about that you don't see during the day. Foxes sneaking through fences, their eyes flashing green from the reflection of my car headlights. A deer flying over a hedge as if it had invisible wings. A massive badger bumbling along. I was the first to arrive and it suddenly felt quite creepy.

Oh heck, I don't like this, I worried silently. *I'll wait for Jack. Or should I just get out? What to do? I don't want to sit here on my own either! Someone might sneak up and get in the car! Shit, I'll open the gate.*

I gingerly stepped out of my car and looked around in the dark with my eyes wide, searching to see if anything or anyone was there. I couldn't see anything so I tiptoed over to unlock the gate, which wasn't very easy in the dark.

I can't see! I need a torch. Where's my phone? Don't tell me I haven't brought it. Oh my God, what if I get murdered?

'Evenin',' a man's voice made my heart explode with fear. I looked round to find a very tall, stocky young man looming over me, holding a rifle. I was frozen. Too terrified to speak.

He's going to kill me! My mind flew into panic mode.

'Don't suppose you'd like me to sort out your rabbit problem?' he asked.

'Er, rabbits?' I squeaked. My throat felt tight and I could feel my heart booming in my chest.

'Yeah you know. They can injure horses' legs if they make too many holes in your field. And actually, it's the law for landowners to control their rabbit population.'

'Really? Er right er I didn't know about that. It's not my land, I just rent it.' I felt sick.

What the hell sort of weird question is that? What does he want? Where is Jack? My mind screamed.

'Yeah, I know who owns it. He's never bothered to sort out his rabbits but it's actually your legal responsibility to sort the rabbits now because you rent it. And the ragwort. You've got loads in there and that's against the law too.'

'How do you know about the ragwort in there?'

'I go in to pick up the birds I shoot,' he replied.

'Oh! It's you!' I gasped, no longer afraid. 'You're the guy who was shooting when we were out riding! You shot me near my eye, you bloody idiot!' I was furious to finally meet the bird shooter.

'Nah, that wasn't me! But I know which dickhead it was. I'm Rob,' he offered his hand, and unthinking I shook it. 'I always stop when I see riders or walkers. I work for the Deerwood Estate so I do things properly.'

'Oh ok. I'm Grace,' I replied. 'So who was shooting when we were riding?'

'That'll be Len. He's a poacher and a right pain in the arse. He's stole a load of my mole traps last week, the bastard. You'll need to make sure your moles don't get out of hand too. They can damage horses' legs as well.'

'Oh hell. That's too much to think about.' The more Rob talked, the more inadequate I felt to be in charge of land maintenance.

'I can sort it all for you, if you like?' asked Rob.

'Could you? Will it be expensive?' I was dreading how much it would cost.

'No, it'll be nothing. I get paid by the estate and the estate owns the shooting rights on this field so it's fine. I only wanted to get an agreement with the landowner or tenant to come on and do it. I like to do things politely because actually I could come on here anyway.' My mind was thoroughly boggled by all the ins and outs of shooting, a subject I'd never had anything to do with.

'Thank you, that's great.' I was very relieved and Rob seemed like a nice guy. I'd almost forgotten why I was even there at night when suddenly car headlights down the lane reminded me what I was doing. Jack pulled into the layby.

'Right, I'll be off. I'm hoping to catch Len up to no good.' Rob winked and disappeared into the night without even asking why I was there in the dark. Being out in the black of night was obviously a really ordinary thing for him.

'Who was that?' asked Jack when she got out of her van.

'He's the gamekeeper from the estate. Not the idiot who shot us all the other week. He's called Rob and he said he's going to sort out the rabbits and the moles for us for free!'

'Great! Wish he could sort out the bloody ragwort too while he's at it,' sighed Jack. Just then a bright light startled us. It was Gillian. She was riding a bicycle and when she dismounted, we could see that she was wearing what appeared to be a mediaeval style gown.

'Isn't it a glorious evening to cast spells?' she trilled as she leaned her bike against the fence in our carpark. Jack and I nodded dumbly. 'I've dressed for the occasion as I feel it helps create the mood, don't you agree?'

'Er oh, how lovely!' was all I could muster in response.

'Now then, ladies, here is the homeopathic preparation of your ragwort, which I made earlier.' Gillian took a fancy glass bottle out of her rucksack and gave it a good shake. It was very small and I wondered how she was going to cover the whole field with it.

'What do we do now?' asked Jack with a hint of embarrassed impatience. Gillian rummaged around in the rucksack again and pulled out an ancient and very dilapidated book.

'The farmer's almanac from times past.' She flourished the book dramatically and with the light of a head torch, she flicked through until she found the page she was looking for.

'First, we must walk the entire perimeter of the land in total silence to clarify the boundary,' she read. 'Absolutely no talking whatsoever.'

'Ok let's get on with it,' said Jack. I smothered a laugh by turning it into a cough. It was reminding me of how irritated Jack used to get with Alex, but this was madder than anything Alex had ever suggested. By the light of the moon and the stars, we walked around the edge of the entire field. Everything looked different in the dark. The horses were like giant, ethereal shadows, looming over us with heightened interest, clearly wondering what the hell we were doing. Everything sounded louder than normal too. The grass seemed to crunch under foot and the light wind in the branches of the Hawthorne, gently rustled the leaves sounding like sandpaper.

'Bloody hell,' muttered Jack as she stumbled over a rabbit burrow. Gillian shot her a look as I stifled the urge to guffaw. Luckily it was right at the very end of the walk round so Gillian let it pass. She opened the book and peered at the page, muttering incoherently as she read. Jack looked at me and raised an eyebrow. I had to bite my lip to control myself.

'Ah. Now it says we must stand in the middle of the field and offer the incantation to the nature spirits,' said Gillian, very matter-of-factly.

'The what?' spluttered Jack.

'The nature spirits,' repeated Gillian. 'I suppose they are like the fairy folk who are said to assist the growth of nature.'

'Right,' said Jack. I was almost at bursting point looking at Jack's face. I had to look away and start thinking about shopping lists to calm myself down. I daren't let Jack know that I had always had a secret interest in this sort of thing. I'd been reading about how some people got 'in tune' with nature spirits and they managed to grow enormous vegetables and I found it a fascinating concept.

Gillian led the way into the middle of the field, shone her head torch on her rucksack and pulled out a large, wooden recorder. 'I will begin by offering the nature spirits some soul music,' she said earnestly. Jack's jaw dropped open while I was rendered speechless as Gillian began to play Greensleeves. It was actually quite beautiful to hear the haunting melody under the full moon but I could see that Jack's brain was not coping very well with this and I was dying to laugh at her expression alone. The musical recital finished and Gillian put the recorder away and read the next part of the ritual. She cleared her throat and studied the book.

'Mother Nature, the creator of life and harmony. Bring back ye balance to thine land. Rid this earth of insert the name of the plant you wish to clear. Oh whoops! I should have said ragwort gosh I am a silly! Rid this earth of ragwort now and for evermore. We give thanks to the pull of the moon and the – oh that's another incantation. Ha! Right let me see, what do we do next?' Gillian squinted at the page. Jack rolled her eyes heavenward while I grinned inanely. I was thoroughly enjoying the whole mad proceedings.

'Oh now we have to sprinkle the remedy on the earth.' She opened the bottle and unfortunately dropped it. It landed on a poo. 'Oh goodness oopsy daisy!' Gillian swiftly grabbed the bottle, wiped the poo from her hand onto her dress and poured out what was left onto the ground.

'Is that it?' asked Jack, losing the last thread of her patience.

'I do believe it is! That was fun wasn't it? Well do let me know how you get on. I'll pop over another day.' And with that, Gillian gathered up her billowing skirts and marched over to the carpark, got on her bike and cycled away into the night.

'Christ almighty,' sighed Jack, wiping her sleeve across her forehead. 'I can't believe we just did that for a bloody weed!'

I exploded with laughter. Tears streaming down my cheeks.

'I don't think that's gonna get rid of your ragwort, ladies,' laughed a familiar voice nearby. We both jumped out of our skins as Rob the gamekeeper appeared out of the darkness. I introduced him to Jack. 'I was watching that. Much better than tv!'

'We don't normally do things like that,' explained Jack with embarrassment.

'Well she said it worked for her ragwort, so we thought it was worth a go,' I laughed.

'She won't get any ragwort in her field,' smirked Rob. 'Her husband is a sheep farmer. Sheep eat ragwort!'

'Oh for God's sake,' Jack erupted with exasperation.

'You need to spray it,' said Rob.

'What with? It can't be anything toxic, we've got horses,' I replied.

'Dunno. A flame thrower? I'd best be off, I've got a fox to catch. Good night, ladies, and thanks for the entertainment,' Rob chuckled and disappeared back into the darkness.

'He's no help,' muttered Jack. 'And we still don't know what to do about this flipping ragwort.'

'Yes, but at least we had a bit of fun,' I laughed. 'God I really needed that. You couldn't make it up could you?'

'No,' laughed Jack. 'I suppose it was funny in hindsight but let's never mention it to anyone or the men in white coats will come to take us away.'

I drove home laughing and became aware of a new sense of belonging. Almost as if meeting a few of the locals had embedded me into that part of Yorkshire, even though I didn't live there. It was a very pleasant sensation.

Chapter 15

'I've had an idea!' texted Jack early one morning as I was feeding Wrexford and mentally preparing for work.

Oh God not again. What the hell is she going to do now? My mind went into panic mode.

'Do I dare ask what it is?' I replied, and then my phone began ringing.

'Couldn't be bothered to text,' laughed Jack. 'Right here's my idea, you'll love it!'

'Hmm, go on.' I doubted I'd love whatever she was going to suggest.

'How about we take a horse on full livery? Because that will pay for our rent!' Jack enthused. I was stunned by the concept. It actually sounded like a brilliant plan.

'That's a good idea!' I responded. 'But what do you mean by full livery? We don't have stables.'

'We would do the extra shit shovelling in the field and feed and do rug stuff if it needed it. I was thinking we could ask Sapna. Remember her saying she wished she was still at our field?'

'God yes, she did say that didn't she? That's not a bad idea. Let's chat about it later. I'll be there around four after school pickup. Florence wants to see Maverick and Toffee.'

'Ok fab, see you then!'

Although the extra shit shovelling felt like a big burden that I didn't have time for, the thought of covering our field rent sounded like a terrific idea and would give me spare money to spend on the dreaded ragwort. Unfortunately, I still had no idea what to actually do about the ragwort. The day passed in a haze of housework and massage work and suddenly it was school pickup time again.

'Are we going to see Toffee and Maverick?' asked Florence, full of enthusiasm.

'We are,' I replied. It was so lovely to see how excited she was about going to see the ponies. It reminded me of how excited I felt every Saturday morning before my weekly riding lesson. It was the highlight of my entire life.

The field gate was open when I arrived so I had the luxury of driving straight into the carpark without having to stop and unlock it first. I thought wistfully about electric gates but I knew that wasn't going to be an option.

'Ay up, Flo!' greeted Jack as Florence bounded over to her. 'Are you going to ride Maverick for me again today?'

'Yay!' said Florence, bursting with excitement.

'Let's get some more photos and videos,' said Jack pulling her camera out of her pocket. Luckily Maverick was in a quiet mood so Florence went to get him herself. Watching her go into his pen with a headcollar made my heart burst into 'rainbows and unicorns'. How I'd longed to be able to do such a thing at her age. It was a wonderful thing to be able to watch my own daughter living my childhood dream. Maverick was such a great little pony and it was a bit sad to have no idea of his history. He'd obviously been very well cared for and well trained because he did walk, trot and canter perfectly and Jack was able to get some excellent videos. It was just a shame about his unsavoury habit that let him down and that was probably the reason why he had ended up at the livestock auction.

'Great stuff, Flo,' smiled Jack as Florence brought Maverick to a smooth halt. 'You're a grand little rider!'

'Think Like a Pony teach me how to ride properly,' said Florence, full of pride for her riding school.

'I can tell,' nodded Jack. 'Wish I'd learned to ride like that.'

'Me too,' I agreed, remembering how harsh my early riding instructors had been.

'Right, you untack him and then put him back in his pen while I chat with your ma.' Jack smiled. She was such a natural with kids. 'Then you can go and give Toffee a groom if you like?' Florence got on with her tasks and Jack and I leaned on the fence to talk about her idea.

'So as it happens, I bumped into Sapna earlier in a sandwich shop,' began Jack. 'She said she'd love to come back here because she can't ride Velvet any more.'

'Really? That's a shame. Why can't she ride her any more?'

'Something to do with an old tendon injury that flared up again. Can't remember what she said exactly but the vet said she can go out in hand but not be ridden.'

'Oh that's so sad!'

'Yeah but she's quite an old horse.'

'Is she? She doesn't look it. How old is she?'

'I think she said around twenty. Bummer isn't it? Anyway, she agreed to paying us a hundred and fifty a month to keep her here.'

'Wow! That's more than what we're paying though. Is it ok to do that?'

'Yes,' grinned Jack, 'because we're doing all the hard work, plus it will cover the cost of winter hay and maybe some maintenance.'

'Ah yes good point, I'd not thought of that,' I replied. I was elated at the thought of not having to pay any more rent. That would make James very happy indeed as it was certainly a big expense to own a horse. 'Brilliant! Thanks so much for sorting that. What's the plan? When will she move her over?'

'I've not actually discussed that bit, to be honest, so I don't know. I'll call her later. But I think she'll want to come fairly soon.'

'Hello ladies! Isn't it a lovely day?' boomed the voice of our landlord behind us suddenly. I jumped out of my skin.

'Oh hello,' I replied, weakly. Dreading what he was going to say about Toffee and Maverick.

'I've bought some apples for the horses.' He handed me the bag and with that he turned and walked off.

'What the heck just happened then?' asked Jack. She was as shocked as I was. 'Those apples are from Waitrose!' I looked at the bag and saw that they were indeed Pink Lady apples from Waitrose.

'How bizarre,' I said. 'I can't believe he didn't say anything about the ponies.'

'I know! I thought we were in for it then. I wasn't expecting apples. Never mind the horses, I'm having one myself.'

We both had an apple and gave the rest to the horses, then Florence and I got in the car to leave. All the way home, Florence was singing a song she'd made up about Toffee. It was very cute but it made me feel stressed as it appeared she believed that Toffee was going to end up being her pony. It wasn't just the extra expense of having a pony, it was the reality of the fact that she might one day grow out of her. We didn't have a clue how big Toffee was going to end up and I assumed that Florence would be taller than me eventually.

During the evening I spent many miserable hours Googling ragwort and learning all about how it's one of the toughest and most invasive poisonous weeds. It made for very depressing reading. The law said that it had to be controlled and carefully disposed of and that the responsibility fell to the person using the land so there was no point even thinking about involving our mercurial landlord, who would no doubt give us short shrift. Suddenly, my eye fell on a website entitled the Ragwort Man and there was a phone number to call for advice. I was feeling so desperate, I rang the number immediately.

'Hello?' I was surprised to be greeted by a terribly posh voice. For some reason I was expecting to hear a thick, Yorkshire accent.

'Hello!' I replied. 'Are you the ragwort man?'

'I am yes. How may I be of assistance?' He sounded so kind I almost cried.

'I've just started renting a field and it's full of ragwort and I have no idea how to deal with it!'

'Oh dear. That's not very good is it? Can you tell me how much land you're renting?'

'It's about seven acres or is it six? Something like that anyway.'

'I see. And can you tell me what the concentration of ragwort is per square metre? How many plants have you noticed?'

'Oh my God, absolutely loads, and they keep popping up every day! It's like a bad dream!'

'Oh dear, that's rather a lot isn't it? Now can you tell me, are you grazing horses and any other animals on the land?'

'Yes, just horses,' I sighed.

'Oh dear. You'll need to remove them asap really,' said the Ragwort Man, which wasn't very helpful.

'We can't move them! We've got nowhere else to go!'

'Oh dear. Well, you'll have to get rid of the ragwort as soon as you can.'

'Well yes.' I was beginning to feel slightly irritated. This wasn't the sort of conversation I had in mind. I was expecting advice. 'But I don't know how to get rid of it!'

'Ah well, there are a number of methods. The best solution would be to get hold of the tansy ragwort flea beetle. Have you heard of it?'

'No. What is it?'

'It's a marvellous little fellow. Absolutely tiny! About the size of your little finger nail so it's a drat to try to find them. Anyway, the grub eats the roots of the ragwort plant while the adult eats the rest of the plant. It's the perfect solution!'

'Wow that's amazing, how perfect!' Relief enveloped me like a warm fluffy blanket. 'Where can I get some?'

'Ah well that's the problem. You can't. They're a protected species and they don't seem to live very well in this country. They prefer the Mediterranean climate.'

'Oh no!' My hopes dashed to the ground. 'What other methods are there?'

'Well now, there is the cinnabar moth. It's red and black so you can't miss it. It loves to eat ragwort and it flourishes here in the UK.'

'Oh great, what a relief!' I whooped with joy. 'Where can I get some?'

'Oh good heavens no no no. You don't want to use the cinnabar moth in a grazing pasture!' exclaimed the Ragwort Man as if I had suggested setting fire to the field.

'Why? You just said it eats ragwort!' I was confused.

'Yes, it eats the plant, which then of course triggers the roots to spread and create even more ragwort plants! Do not under any circumstances allow the cinnabar moth into your field. It is only useful to control ragwort in the hedgerows.'

'So what can I do?' I cried, almost at breaking point.

'Well,' sighed the Ragwort Man. 'You could try spraying it with Verdone.'

'Is that expensive?' I hardly dare ask.

'No it's very cheap,' he replied.

'Oh great! Is it toxic though?' I was very wary of spraying anything.

'Oh yes! It's terrible stuff and it will kill all the grass too. You don't want to use that in a grazing pasture, good heavens no.'

'Well is there anything you can suggest that won't kill all the grass?' My chest was feeling tight and my heart rate had increased ten-fold.

'Yes indeed! There is a powerful chemical 2,4-D, which is in a few commercial sprays. This will kill all of your ragwort and it's quite inexpensive. You would need to pay someone with a tractor to spray it, though and it must be applied while the plant is in the rosette stage as it is a growth inhibitor so it won't work on fully grown ragwort plants. Of course, it will kill absolutely every other broad leaf plant in your field but the grass will remain.' I had given up caring about all the other plants. I just wanted rid of the ragwort and this sounded like a great solution.

'That sounds good,' I said.

'Hmm well, I wouldn't use it in my own grazing pasture.'

'Oh? Why not?'

'Would you want to spray anything toxic on the ground where your beloved horses graze? Good heavens! It's awful stuff and I have noticed that more cases of laminitis are triggered when horses graze on pasture sprayed with that dreadful chemical. Avoid it like the plague!'

'Oh for God's sake! I thought you were going to tell me how to solve this! It just seems like a worse problem now!' I finally flipped.

'Oh dear, oh dear. Panic not! There is a perfectly healthy and effective solution.'

'Really?' I didn't dare to feel hopeful.

'Yes. It's called citronella. Have you heard of it?'

'The lemon-scented oil?' I couldn't believe my ears and assumed he was raving mad.

'That's right yes!' he enthused. 'Now this particular oil kills ragwort to the root and is perfectly safe for horses to graze where it has been sprayed. Do you have a computer to hand? If so, Google it now while we are on the phone together.'

'Er, yes I have. Hang on a minute,' I reached over to my laptop and googled citronella and ragwort. I was expecting to see absolutely nothing but my eyes popped out of my head when I saw that it actually does kill ragwort to the root at any stage of the growing phase and that it's non-toxic and safe for horses.

'Wow!' I almost shouted. 'You're right!'

'There now! Isn't that a relief?' chuckled the Ragwort Man.

'Yes it is! But how do I use it? Do I need a tractor?'

'No, you need to be very careful to only spray the ragwort or all the grass will taste revolting. You will need to buy a good five to ten litres of pure citronella, dilute it in water to thirty-three percent and add a coloured marker dye so you can see where you've already sprayed. Then, using a knapsack sprayer just walk round the field and hand-spray what you can see. You'll soon get it under control after a year or so, so don't panic too much. And, of course, the delightful aroma will keep the flies away from your field! Good luck and cheerio!' The Ragwort Man hung up and I breathed a deep sigh of relief. As an aromatherapist I had a great contact who would give me gallons of citronella for next to nothing. I just had to get a knapsack sprayer and some dye.

For the first time in a long time, I slept soundly without any awful nightmares about ragwort and awoke the following morning feeling refreshed. After school drop off and dog walk, I decided to go to the field and do a bit of schooling with Poppy.

'Oh wow!' I said out loud as I noticed Adam the farmer spraying weeds on the side of the road using a knapsack sprayer. I wound my window down.

'Hi Adam!' Adam stopped spraying and smiled warmly.

'Now then,' he greeted. 'I'm just getting rid of these thistles. Can't stand the buggers getting into my pastures. Ruins everything you know.'

'Would it be possible to borrow your knapsack sprayer? I need to spray our ragwort,' I asked.

'Oh aye. Your landlord never bothered with ragwort. I'm glad to hear you're going to sort it out. You can come and get it tomorrow when I've finished. I'll leave it in my yard by the tap. You know ragwort is very poisonous so mek sure you're wearing ...' I never got to hear the rest of his sentence because he walked off, spraying the weeds as he went and then hopped over the wall into his field and waved goodbye.

'How odd,' I laughed and continued driving to our field. I pulled over, got out of the car and stretched. It was a gloriously warm spring day, the hawthorn hedges had finally burst into their fluffy white blossom and looked like a wedding ceremony. The sweet, heady aroma was intoxicating and I was really looking forward to using the school with Poppy.

'Oh my God!' I exclaimed as I opened the gate. Maverick had knocked Valerie over, escaped his pen and was busy humping Toffee, who was standing quite happily allowing him to do it while Poppy looked on aghast. Buddy shot me a look and snorted. If he could have spoken, I'm sure he would have said 'Disgusting!' or something similar.

'Maverick! Stop it!' I shouted, running over to him and waving my arms around. Maverick galloped off squealing and Toffee came over for a cuddle. I say cuddle in the loosest sense of the word. She actually came over, bashed her head into my chest and started pushing into me, almost knocking me over. She was a lovable pest but what to do about Maverick, who was eyeing up Poppy? Poppy gave him 'bugger off' signals but it didn't deter him in the slightest. He bravely strutted over to her and attempted to mount. Poppy gave him both barrels, booting him in his head and then she galloped off.

'Well it serves you right,' I said to the stunned Maverick, who was clearly seeing stars. 'Maybe that will teach you to leave her alone?' I felt quite doubtful but hoped it might help.

'Er excuse me?' called a voice from the carpark. I looked over and saw a middle-aged man and woman both wearing hiking gear. 'Is that horse ok?' I walked over to them.

'Yes he's fine. He needs to learn to leave the ladies alone,' I laughed.

'Well he doesn't look fine to me,' snapped the man. 'He's been lying like that since we walked past three hours ago and I know for a fact that horses don't lie down for that long!'

'What?' I had no idea what the man was talking about.

'That horse over there!' the increasingly annoyed man pointed over to Valerie, lying forlornly on her side with all her legs sticking out.

'Oh! That's just Valerie. Maverick knocked her over,' I laughed.

'I don't see what's so amusing about that. She looks like she's dead to me.' The man looked horrified.

'Yeah I suppose she does look like she's dead,' I agreed.

'Well don't you think you should be calling for a vet?' demanded the woman, giving me the dirtiest stare I'd ever received.

'No? Why would I do that? We'll move her out of the way later.'

'Barbara dear, call the RSPCA immediately,' snarled the man as he leaped over our fence and marched towards the prone Valerie. I was stunned. The woman pulled her phone out of her pocket and started Googling the RSPCA.

'People like you shouldn't have animals,' she spat.

'Pardon?' I couldn't believe my ears and walked after the man who had reached Valerie.

'Oh!' he said. 'It's not real!'

'What? Could you not tell?' I was gobsmacked.

'No, I thought it was a dead horse! Gosh, I must apologise for being so angry!' the man's face was beet red.

'That's ok,' I laughed. 'The lady who made it will be very happy to hear that it was good enough to fool you.'

'Oh goodness,' said the woman who had come over the fence to look. 'I am so sorry I was so rude!' She looked horrified. 'I thought you were an animal abuser!'

'Not to worry! It's all very funny in hindsight. I didn't know what you were talking about. I thought you were both mad.' I laughed my head off which made them laugh, and they took some photos to tell their friends and went on their way.

When I'd recovered my composure, I lifted the heavy Valerie to her feet so that nobody else would think we had a dead horse in the field and then I took Maverick's pen down, as it seemed pointless keeping it up.

'You are going to have to get a new home asap,' I said as he trotted past me. It was a shame because he was stunning and Florence could ride him, and if we'd had the money and if he wasn't such a sex pest I would have kept him. But the reality was we couldn't keep him so I phoned Jack to tell her he'd escaped and I told her about the dead Valerie incident, which she found hilarious.

'The advert has already attracted someone and she's coming to see him tomorrow afternoon,' said Jack.

'That's a relief,' I replied. 'Let's hope she wants him.'

'Yes, fingers crossed for that.'

Chapter 16

The following day couldn't come soon enough. My mind had gone into overdrive about the ragwort during the night and I was on tenterhooks hoping that the citronella would work. I just needed to get the knapsack sprayer and hoped Adam had remembered to leave it outside for me. I was also worrying about Maverick and whether or not his obscene behaviour would put off potential buyers. If it did what would we do? I didn't like to think of him ending up at the sales again. He could end up somewhere awful. I tried to put it all out of my mind while I got Florence ready for school and sorted out Wrexford. By the time I was able to set off to the field, my heart was doing a tap dance in my chest.

I pulled into Adam's farmyard and stepped out of the car. It was very clean and well kept. The sheep dog was lying nearby in a kennel, chewing on a thick stick and wasn't remotely concerned that I was there. In a large wire pen next to the kennel was a very waggy tailed German Shepherd. **'Beware of the dog!'** read a sign on the door of his pen.

'You're not much of a guard dog are you?' I laughed as the dog pranced around with a squeaky toy in his mouth, desperate to say hello. A sudden onslaught of ferocious barking behind me made me jump out of my skin. I turned to find Wendy's mother-in-law being pulled out of her house by a black Labrador with bared teeth going absolutely crazy.

'Tulip! Stop it!' she shouted, but to no avail. She had to pull with both hands on the lead to keep the enraged Tulip from attacking me. I was frozen to the spot having never experienced a Labrador like that. Fortunately, Adam came hurtling over from a nearby barn, grabbed Tulip and told her to shut up. It worked.

'Go and tek her in back field for a walk,' he said to his wife. She muttered something under her breath and walked haughtily off with the dog.

'Sorry about that. We don't quite know why that 'un's a bit mental like. And that 'un's as soft as butter.' He gestured to the German Shepherd. 'And the sheep dog's neither use nor ornament neither.' He shrugged. 'Never mind. You'll be wanting the knapsack I s'pose?'

'Yes please,' I replied.

'Aye, it's over here.' Adam led me across the yard to where he'd left the sprayer.

'This is a lovely farm,' I sighed wistfully. 'I wish I could own a place like this.'

'I was born in the house here.' Adam nodded. 'And I left school at fourteen to help mi dad. There were a lot more people living here when I were young but then Yorkshire water made a compulsory purchase order on the whole village and we had to fight to ... anyway I must get on. Cheerio!' and off he went.

'And that's why we call him *Half-a-story Adam*,' laughed Wendy, who had just driven into the yard. 'I've still to hear the rest of that story too.'

'He always walks away in mid-sentence. It's so bizarre.'

'You get used to him eventually. What are you spraying?' Wendy nodded at the sprayer.

'Ragwort.' I grimaced. 'It's been stressing me out!'

'Oh good luck. It's a bugger isn't it? I need to sort mine out.

It's popping up all over in Denwyn's paddock. Let me know how you get on with it.'

In the boot of my car, I had an enormous container of citronella that'd I'd been lucky enough to get at a very reasonable price. The aroma was so pungent though, I could taste it and it was very sickly. However, if it worked that would be amazing. I measured it out at least four times just to be absolutely certain I'd got it right and then topped up the sprayer with water and added some blue dye. It was at that moment when I realised how heavy water is. I was shocked at how hard it was to heave the sprayer onto my back.

'Do you need a hand?' I jumped. Roger, the landlord, was in his garden watching my struggles.

'Er well that would be kind if you're not too busy?' I squirmed.

'No I'm not busy right now. I'd be delighted to help.' Roger hopped over the gate into the field.

Oh my God how weird! Why is he suddenly being so nice? My mind was perturbed. I had no idea how to respond to this unusually friendly side of Roger.

'What are you doing?' he asked looking genuinely interested.

'I was attempting to spray the ragwort because it's taking over the entire field but I didn't realise how heavy this knapsack would be,' I explained.

'No problem,' replied Roger as he picked up the knapsack sprayer as if it weighed nothing. 'So where is this ragwort and why are you spraying it?

'This is ragwort!' I said, pointing at a fat rosette, astonished by his question. 'It's a poisonous plant that destroys the liver and eventually kills the animals that eat it. Did you not know?'

'Well, I had sort of heard Adam complaining about it but I'm too busy to deal with weeds. I didn't know it could kill. That's no good is it?'

'It's no good at all, and it's actually the law to remove it from your land and you've got loads and loads of it!'

'Oh well it's a good job we're doing it then isn't it?'

'Yes,' I sighed. I was annoyed that I was having to waste my time spraying someone else's land, who clearly couldn't care less about it, when I had hardly any spare time to ride my horse.

'You know, when I bought this house, I had dreams of becoming a farmer,' said Roger wistfully.

'Really? That's surprising. What sort of farming?' I couldn't imagine Roger doing anything of the sort.

'Well at first, I thought, I'll get some rare breed pigs but Valentina couldn't cope with the smell so we scrapped that idea. Then I fancied getting some Aberdeen Angus cattle but it's a lot of work looking after animals and I'm a busy man so I dropped that plan.'

'It's a shame to have all this land and not use it yourself.'

'Yes it is a bit, but I love making money. You can't make a lot of money out of farming can you?'

'No but you can get a lot of happiness just from being with animals.' I was stunned by his attitude and glad that I wasn't like that.

'I suppose so. I like seeing your horses and not having to look after them myself so that's enough for me,' laughed Roger. 'This stuff smells of citronella, doesn't it?'

'That's because it is citronella! It kills ragwort. I don't know how but apparently it does so fingers crossed it works.'

We walked round the field spraying ragwort for a good two hours, while Roger regaled me with stories of his youth. It was interesting to get to know him and he seemed like such a nice man – the total opposite of how he had appeared to be. It was very odd. Then he had to get back to work, which was actually a relief because I couldn't stand the smell of citronella any more and my mind couldn't cope with this new nice Roger. As he walked away, I realised that his love of money was probably what made him so cross and I felt quite sorry for him. I looked around at the beauty of the field. Every inch of it had burst into new life from the hedgerows covered in may flowers to the deep green banks of nettles and fluffy purple thistles. Dandelions were popping up all over, which the horses loved to eat, and delicate daisies decorated the top half of the field, but not the bottom, which I found bizarre. The ragwort looked quite comical with large patches of blue all over it and I was pleased to see it was already beginning to shrivel up. I was also covered in blue dye and looked like a smurf. I had no idea how I'd managed to get it all over me.

'I like your blue legs,' laughed Rob, who was leaning over our carpark fence. 'I got a few of your rabbits last night you'll be glad to know.' He lifted up a bag that looked quite full.

'Oh the poor things.' I felt very sad for them.

'Yeah, well what can we do? Mankind has ruined the balance of nature so people like me have to sort it out and we get loads of grief for it.'

'I hadn't thought of it that way,' I replied.

'People are always telling me off for shooting but if I didn't do it, we'd have no crops in those fields.'

'True.' I nodded.

'You should come with me some time and I'll show you what goes on after dark.' Rob smiled.

'That would be interesting! I'm not sure what my husband would think of me hanging out with a young man in the dark though.'

'I'm not interested in women.' Rob winked. 'I might like your husband though.'

'Oh!' I was relieved to hear that. 'Fab, then yes I'd be very interested to see the wildlife round here at night.'

'Great, here's my number so just text me when you want to meet. I'm out pretty much every night.' Rob gave me a business card and then went on his way.

I looked at my watch and realised I needed to head off home and do a few boring things before school pickup time. I wanted to be at the field to help Jack with Maverick when the lady came to see him. It was very frustrating to have no time for Poppy though. Having our own land was turning out to be much more time consuming than I had imagined. I sighed, got into the car and set off.

Jack was busy grooming Maverick when I returned to the field in the afternoon and Florence was with me in case the lady wanted to see him being ridden.

'I hope she turns up,' said Jack, stretching her back. 'I've been grooming him for ages.'

'I can tell. Have you used some optical brighteners on him? He's so clean it's hurting my eyes.'

'Er actually yes I have.' Jack showed me a bottle of dog shampoo that she'd washed him with and it was for showing white dogs. 'I used the whole bottle! Took me ages to rinse it off!'

'Well we all need sunglasses to look at him now.'

'Poor Maverick, he doesn't want to be sold,' said Florence sadly.

'He does,' I replied. 'He wants to be in a lovely kind home with someone who can ride him every day.'

'I could ride him every day,' replied Florence with a very hopeful expression on her face. I felt awful having to burst her bubble but we couldn't keep Maverick. Fortunately, the lady arrived just at that moment so I was rescued from having to reply.

'Hello!' greeted Jack with great relief. 'Are you Linda?'

'Hello, yes I am. Is this the pony?' asked Linda. She had dwarfism and was the perfect size for Maverick.

'Yes, this is Maverick. Would you like to see him in action?' replied Jack.

'That would be great.' She smiled.

I suddenly felt a surge of anxiety as Jack tacked him up and Florence led him into the school. Luckily, he behaved beautifully and went through his paces with perfection.

'He looks great.' Linda nodded. 'Can I try him?'

Florence jumped off and Linda led Maverick round the arena, talking to him. It was very nice to see how she bothered to make an effort to do that first. Jack looked very impressed. We held our breaths as she mounted, expecting disaster to happen, but Maverick was very relaxed and walked, trotted and cantered without putting a hoof wrong.

'I like him.' Linda grinned as she halted next to us and dismounted. 'Can you tell me about his history?'

'Well, I don't really know because I bought him from the sales not so long ago. Since then he's been ridden by Florence and she's done a great job with him,' replied Jack as Florence untacked

Maverick and turned him loose. 'In his passport there are two previous owners that might be able to tell you more about him if you contact them,' continued Jack leafing through Maverick's passport to show Linda.

'Oh ok that's a good idea.' She nodded. 'What's he been like in general since he's been here?'

'Er, well,' said Jack going red in the face.

'Oh look at Maverick!' shrieked Florence suddenly. 'He's trying to put his willy in Toffee's bottom again!' She roared with laughter and ran over to him, waving her arms about and telling him to stop.

'Yeah so er, that's what I was going to tell you about,' sighed Jack absolutely mortified. Linda stared open mouthed at Maverick humping Toffee while Florence smacked his bottom and shooed him away. 'He's got a thing for the ladies.'

Linda was silent for what felt like an eternity and I held my breath waiting for the inevitable reply.

'Ha! He's a character isn't he?' She suddenly burst out laughing. Her whole body shook and tears began streaming down her cheeks. Jack and I had been so uptight about Maverick that we had been completely unable to see the funny side of his behaviour until now. We both erupted into deep belly laughter and Florence joined us in our mirth until we could all laugh no more. It was a tremendous relief.

'Oh dear!' sighed Linda, wiping her tears. 'I haven't laughed like that for years! You know, I actually don't mind about his humping problem. I feel he's the right pony for me and he'll be in a field with geldings so I'm sure I won't have any trouble.'

Jack and I simultaneously breathed a huge sigh and almost fell over from the shock.

'Oh thank God for that,' said Jack. 'He's a great little guy otherwise!'

'Yes I can see he is and there's no malice in him so I'll have him.' Linda smiled, reaching in her pocket and pulling out a huge wad of cash. 'I came prepared because I just knew he would be mine!'

Such a quick decision really surprised me.

'I can come and collect him tomorrow if that's ok?' Linda was so keen, it was the most perfect scenario. She paid the cash and arranged a time to collect him and left Jack and me grinning. Florence was very sad though.

'Don't be sad, Flo,' said Jack. 'You're going to be busy looking after Toffee for me now.'

Florence whooped and ran off to see Toffee, who was busy stripping the bark from a nearby tree for no apparent reason. She wasn't eating it, we could see she was spitting it out.

'She's a mad pony isn't, she?' Jack shook her head.

'She is.' I nodded. 'Thank God about Maverick. I can't believe how easy that was!'

'I know! It was like a miracle. How perfect is Linda? He'll have a home for life with her.'

'Yep. He's a very lucky pony.' I nodded. I couldn't believe that fate had found him a small woman who clearly loved him instantly, despite his terrible behaviour. I was glad he hadn't gone to a child who would outgrow him and sell him on and on and on until he was too old for anyone to want him. The thought made me choke up with tears and I had to pretend I had a fly in my eye.

Driving home, my mind felt very happy and relieved to have one less thing to stress about. A fox darted across the road and jumped through the hedge into a field, which made me ponder on a possible nighttime adventure with Rob learning about the nocturnal wildlife. I definitely wanted to learn more about nature.

Chapter 17

Thanks to the responsibility of land management, I hadn't been able to do any schooling with Poppy for a long time and my mind began to spiral.

Why did we take on a huge field? I haven't got time for this! I just want to turn up, ride and go home. I don't want to spray weeds, shovel shits and constantly mend fences.

You aren't mending any fences, interjected the really sensible part of my brain. *Jack's mending all the fences.*

Yes but I have to sometimes help hold things while she's doing that and it takes up so much time! I replied angrily to myself.

Just then my phone pinged.

'I'm full of snot so I can't come today. I'm so sorry!' texted Lady Alexa, who was due to come in half an hour. Before I had time to reply my phone pinged again

'I've just lost a filling so I need to go to the dentist this morning I'm so sorry!' text the second client of the morning.

'Wow!' I said out loud and whooped. I didn't normally celebrate losing out on a morning's work but I felt so relieved that I would now have time to ride, guilt free because it wasn't my fault they cancelled. I replied sympathetically to both clients, dashed upstairs to change into my jodhpurs and ran out of the house before something boring caught my eye like the washing or cooking and so on. All that could wait.

I sang loudly all the way to the field. It was a gloriously sunny day, almost summer, and the sky was a beautiful deep blue. All the trees were in full leaf and the hedgerows were a riot of

colour thanks to the abundance of wildflowers. I especially loved
the scent of the cow parsley, which was very similar to fennel. I
steeled myself for the possibility that Toffee would be in some sort
of bother when I arrived and almost held my breath as I opened
the gate, not daring to look.

'Toffee!' I yelled. She was in the back field which we had closed
off to grow for a while. It had taken hours of faff to fill in all
the gaps in the hedge with random things like pallets, rope, old
branches and so on. We thought we had done a good job but
clearly we hadn't. Toffee casually looked over at me and then went
back to grazing.

'How the hell did you get in there?' I chuntered. I walked the
entire hedge line but couldn't see how it was possible that she
got in.

'Did you jump the gate?' I asked her, as I slipped her headcollar
on and led her out. She put her nose on me and asked for a head
scratch. 'It's a good job you're cute.' I gave her a scratch and then
turned her loose in the front field and walked off to find Poppy,
who was all the way at the bottom of the field, drinking and
paddling. It was beautiful at the bottom of the field. There were
very large and bizarre grassy mounds that were reminiscent of
some ancient burial grounds and banks of wild flowers. A huge
willow tree bowed over the stream, its feathery branches almost
dancing in the water, which bubbled over the rocks, and it was
hypnotic to watch the long grasses as they waved from side to
side in the current. Poppy lumbered out of the stream and began
marching up the field. I trotted after her and she came to a stop
at the entrance of the school as if she knew that's what I wanted
to do.

It felt quite exciting to prepare to use my own school without having had to book a slot or share it with someone else. It was just me and Poppy. I led her into the shelter and breathed a sigh of relief as I began to groom.

'Toffee! Will you get out of the way?' Toffee seemed fascinated with my grooming kit and poked her head inside. She was standing very close to Poppy, who had her ears flat back, clearly very annoyed. Toffee didn't seem remotely concerned and she pulled a brush out of the bag and hurled it to the other side of the shelter.

'Toffee!' I shouted and pushed on her to move her away. She waited a few moments before walking back and stood even closer to Poppy. Poppy reversed into her and kicked out. It had absolutely no effect whatsoever. Poppy kicked out again. Toffee couldn't care less. I hastily grabbed her head collar and led her away before she ended up dead but the weird thing was that as soon as I turned her loose, she followed me straight back regardless of the furious rage emanating from Poppy. She was completely oblivious to the point where Poppy gave up bothering to react. She snorted and pulled a face and then resigned herself to the presence of Toffee.

Grooming Poppy was now quite challenging as I had to squeeze round Toffee, who kept snuffling in the grooming bag and pulling things out to inspect them. Sometimes she would chew on things and other times she would toss them aside as if the item had offended her. I kept trying to push her away but it never made any difference, she just kept coming back. It was extremely annoying. Finally, Poppy was groomed and tacked up and I managed to get Toffee to move out of the way so I could lead her over to the school. By now I was feeling quite jangled but I was determined to do some training with Poppy.

Toffee followed us and watched with interest like a spectator as we walked around the school and did some circles, figures of eight and a few wonky serpentines. I was amazed at how relaxed and amenable Poppy was. There was no sign of her challenging behaviour and that helped me to relax further, which had the immediate effect of slowing Poppy's walk. It was fascinating. I decided to practise the things I'd learned in Wales so I focussed my mind on the far end of the school and visualised Poppy trotting. Nothing happened. She just kept walking. I visualised it again but still no change from Poppy, who was contentedly meandering along.

'Bloody hell,' I grumbled. 'Why isn't this working? I suppose I can't actually be bothered to trot so it must be me blocking this?' I was too tired to keep trying and then I suddenly spotted Toffee grazing in the back field again.

'What the hell?' I hadn't noticed her leaving so I had no idea how she'd got in again. It was extremely puzzling, not to mention irritating. I hastily untacked Poppy and ran across to the back field to catch Toffee. Once again, I led her through the gate and turned her loose. In front of my eyes, the little bugger sauntered casually down the field and walked straight through the hedge. It was such a narrow gap I hadn't even seen it but it was big enough for little Toffee to slip through without any problem whatsoever. I pulled my phone out of my pocket and called Jack.

'Toffee can walk through the hedge to get into the back field!' I blurted as soon as she answered the phone.

'Oh bloody hell. We need to rest that field. I'll come up as soon as I can and sort it somehow. God she's a pain in the bum,' replied Jack with a deep sigh.

'She's not daft is she?' laughed Rob, who had appeared as if from nowhere, making me jump out of my skin.

'Christ!' I exclaimed. 'How do you keep doing that?'

'What?' asked Rob.

'You're just suddenly there! Like some sort of ninja!'

'Years of hunting, my dear.' He winked. 'Anyway, I just popped in to see if you want to meet tonight. I need to catch a poacher who's up to no good.'

'That sounds a bit scary,' I replied.

'Nah it's just daft old Len, stealing things as usual. I want to catch him at it and he'll be more polite if I'm with a lady.'

'Oh ok it sounds fun. What time?'

'Meet me here at sundown and we'll go from there,' said Rob. 'Right I'd best get on. See you later on.'

The gate clanged open and I looked over to see Jack coming into the field with a load of rope and a pallet.

'I thought I'd better sort it now,' she said. 'I was only round the corner when you rang. Where's she getting in?' I showed her the gap in the hedge.

'Oh heck she's sneaky isn't she?' grumbled Jack, swiftly getting to work pulling on a few branches to fill out the gap and then tying the pallet in place to block it up.

'There!' She smiled. 'That'll keep her out! Let's see what she does now.' I went into the back field and brought Toffee out again and turned her loose. As if butter wouldn't melt in her mouth, she casually trotted down the hedge line to go straight back in but was blocked by the pallet. Toffee looked at us with surprise and a hint of annoyance. She snorted, kicked at the pallet and then sighed. She then trotted off down the field to look for another way in.

'She's a menace,' laughed Jack. 'Oh hello Buddy.' Buddy had come over for a head scratch.

'What's that in his main?' I asked taking a closer look at a strange sort of plait.

'It looks like a braid,' replied Jack peering at it. 'That's weird isn't it?'

'Looks like you've been marked. You need to come and look at this,' said Rob, who had come back over.

'Marked?' I asked. I had no idea what he was talking about but he was walking at top speed towards the shelter. Jack and I had to run to keep up.

'See that?' Rob pointed at three white lines on the side of the shelter. 'And over here too.' He led us to the gate post where there were the same three white lines.

'What is it?' asked Jack and I simultaneously.

'You've been marked by thieves,' replied Rob. 'You need to call the police.'

'Seriously?' I thought he was joking.

'No way,' said Jack. 'Could that be linked with the weird plait in Buddy's mane?'

'I don't know about that,' said Rob. 'That might just be from the wind? But these marks I've seen before. You can't ignore it.'

'Oh good God.' I felt sick. 'What do we do?'

'I'll call Dave, he's the local police for this area and he's a good lad.' Rob pulled out his phone while Jack and I waited in stunned silence. After a brief chat, Rob hung up and said Dave was on his way. In less than fifteen minutes, the police car pulled into our carpark and Rob introduced us and then showed PC Dave the marks.

'Is this for real?' I suddenly felt a bit silly. 'Surely the white lines could be anything?' Jack was looking a bit sceptical too.

'No.' The policeman shook his head. 'I've seen this before. You've been marked for a theft. We can only guess it's your horses or they might think you've got valuable equipment in your field shelter.'

'Oh my God!' I couldn't believe this could be true.

'What do we do?' asked the practical Jack.

'Well unfortunately, we have a vulnerable missing person so we can't spare any officers to keep watch tonight. You'll have to come up and stay hidden and call us if anything happens. We will come immediately but don't approach them,' replied Dave.

'I can't believe this is happening!' I said, I had gone into a bit of shock.

'I'm afraid these things happen more often than you can imagine,' said Dave sadly. His radio started beeping so he had to leave for another job.

'What are we going to do?' I wailed.

'We're going to catch the bastards,' said Jack with her hands on her hips. 'I'm not standing for it!'

'Well, we need to do it safely,' said Rob. 'These people will be dangerous.'

'Yes,' agreed Jack. 'Have you got any suggestions?'

'Have you got different cars you can borrow? They'll probably know yours,' Rob asked.

'Yes, I can use my husband's car,' I replied.

'And I can borrow my dad's,' said Jack.

'Right. I suggest Grace parks up further down the road and keep yourself hidden. And Jack you patrol the lanes in a circuit.

I'll wait in the car with Grace and Jack can call us if she sees anything suspicious. I'll bring my rifle just in case.'

'Bloody hell. This is all sounding a bit Starsky and Hutch.'

'Grace, pick me up at Adam's farmyard when it's dark,' instructed Rob and then he had to get back to his work.

'Is this really happening?' I felt like I was in a weird dream.

'Seems like it is,' laughed Jack nervously. 'Right, I'll get off and I'll text you when I start my patrols!'

I drove home in a daze, feeling sick to the stomach.

What if they take Poppy and abuse her and I never find her again?

They won't take any of them. You will be waiting! replied the calm centre of my brain.

But what if we can't stop them?

The police will come and stop them!

But what if they're too busy with that bloody missing person? Why is somebody missing today when we need the police? Why isn't there enough police? It's ridiculous, the police should be top priority!

My mind churned round and round tying itself in knots, mirroring the incessant churning of my stomach, which was threatening to eject its contents. It was extremely difficult to focus on mum stuff but I couldn't let Florence know anything about it otherwise she would be terrified for Toffee's safety. I felt like I was bursting inside, having to put on a happy face but luckily I'd had years of experience of pretending to be happy so I managed to pull it off. Florence's bedtime couldn't come soon enough and when I could hear she was asleep I dragged James into the kitchen and told him everything.

'What? Are you serious? This is dangerous! You can't go up there and wait on your own!' he said. 'I will come!'

'You can't! You need to stay here with Florence! I need to get going now. I'll be with Rob anyway.'

'I'm not happy about that!' spluttered James. 'Sitting in a car at night with a guy?'

'He's gay!' I replied.

'Oh! That's alright then. You must keep me informed about what's happening though.'

'I will! Bye!' I grabbed my coat, pulled my boots on and dashed out of the house. It felt weird to be driving James's car. It was immaculately clean, unlike my own. My heart was pounding by the time I got to Adam's farmyard but when I pulled in, Rob was nowhere to be seen.

'I got delayed in Huddersfield,' he texted just as I was wondering where he was. 'Long story. Go and park up where I showed you and lock your doors. I'll be with you as soon as I can.'

Oh my God! This is a nightmare! I daren't tell James I was on my own, he would go berserk. But I couldn't risk leaving and the horses getting stolen.

'I'm driving down the lane!' texted Jack. That made me feel a bit better so I headed off to the layby down the lane where I could still see our gate but be far enough away to not cause concern to any thieves. As I pulled in, Jack drove past in her dad's car and waved. I locked the doors and slunk down in the seat to be as hidden as possible.

The darkness felt heavy and foreboding. It didn't help that thick clouds were blocking out the moon and stars so all I could see was a murky sky. I sat there for what felt like hours of nothing happening when I suddenly heard a motorbike approaching from behind me. I kept very still. It stopped outside our gate. My heart burst into a flutter and I held my breath. Then it went on its way. I breathed a sigh of relief. A few minutes later, it was back and again it stopped outside our gate.

Is that them? I wondered, shifting in my seat to get a better view.

The motorbike drove on again. I pulled out my phone to text Jack but she texted me first.

'A bike keeps driving past!' she texted. 'I'm parked up in the hedge near Adam's farm!'

The bike came back but this time with a car. They both stopped outside our gate and two men got out.

Oh my God! I froze. I couldn't breathe.

The two men shone bright flashlights on the gate post and then hopped over the gate.

Call the police! Instructed the sensible part of my brain. My arms had turned to jelly and dialling 999 felt so difficult.

'What's your emergency?' asked the operator. My voice was hoarse with fear as I whispered what was happening.

'Stay in your car!' she commanded. 'Do not approach them! Police are on their way!'

Within minutes, I could hear sirens from all directions. I couldn't believe my eyes. Two police vans and three police cars swooped in as if from nowhere. The motorbike roared to life and sped off with a police car in hot pursuit. The car did a nifty turn and zoomed towards me at top speed, followed by one of the police vans. The rest of the police jumped out of their cars and leaped over our gate. I could hear a lot of shouting.

'What's going on?' Rob banged on my window almost giving me a heart attack. I opened the door and he got in.

'Oh my God!' I squeaked and poured out the tale. Rob jumped

out of the car and we both ran over to the police, who were leaving our field.

'They got away from us but they've been apprehended down the road!' said the policeman. 'You two need to keep out of the way and go home. We will contact you as soon as we have something to tell you.'

'I'm not going home!' I said to Rob as we walked back to the car. 'What if more of them come and take the horses?'

'Unlikely, but I'll wait with you,' he said and we got back in my car. 'Is that Jack?'

Jack pulled up next to us and wound her window down.

'They got them!' She grinned. 'They're in the police van now!'

'Thank God! That was so scary,' I replied. 'They went into our field!'

'Jeez!'

'We're going to wait here a bit longer,' said Rob. 'But I doubt anyone else will come now.'

'Yeah they've been scared off,' agreed Jack and after a bit more of a chat, she drove off for home. After an hour of nothing happening, I felt that it was safe to leave. I was so exhausted by the time I got home that I fell into a deep sleep as soon as my head hit the pillow. But it felt like only seconds later that I awoke with a jolt at the sound of my alarm.

The horses! What if more of them came later and stole them? I leaped out of bed and dragged my clothes on.

'I've walked the dog and I'll take Florence to school,' said James, almost reading my mind. 'I know you'll be wanting to go straight up to the field.' I kissed him and dashed straight out of the house before anyone could stop me and sped to the field.

'What the bloody hell's been going on?' Roger the landlord greeted me by the gate. 'I've had the police here this morning looking for you! They're in your field shelter. You should have told me what was happening, I'd have come out with you.' I was stunned.

'I didn't think you'd want to be bothered,' I replied.

'Why? Of course I'd be bothered about the safety of your horses,' he exclaimed as if I'd suggested he was a heartless man. 'Anyway, the police have some news for you.' We walked into the shelter where the two police officers were patting the horses.

'Are you Grace?' asked one of them.

'Yes! What happened?' I asked.

'Well, we apprehended them and they had a camera in their possession. We examined it and discovered they had been photographing you and your horse all week. They had also taken several photos of the neighbouring farmyard.'

'No way! Why? That's so creepy!' I felt very disturbed.

'Yes it's disgusting. But the bad news is we couldn't arrest them as we didn't get them on your land. We caught them on the road. They said they hadn't been in your field and we had no proof that it was them who we had chased unfortunately.'

'What?' I couldn't believe my ears. 'But what about the photos?'

'Again, it's not an offence. They said they are "nature watchers" and unfortunately, they can get away with it. But they won't be back here in a hurry. We told them we know they were planning to do a robbery and that we will be keeping a close eye on them.'

'But what if they do come back?' I was furious.

'They won't! Not after the talking to we gave them. Don't

worry.' The policeman gave me a knowing look as if to infer they had scared the living daylights out of them and that helped to ease my worries.

'If it happens again you need to let me know. I want to be involved,' insisted Roger. It was bizarre to see a new caring side to him.

'Er, ok. Thanks, Roger,' I mumbled. Rob arrived at that moment and Roger had to go to work, as did the police.

'Well that wasn't quite the night we had planned was it?' he laughed. 'I'm glad it all got sorted and no horses got stolen.'

'Yes, thank heavens. That was hideous,' I replied.

'I'll be round here most nights so try not to worry too much. And if you want to come and meet me just drop me a text.' Rob winked and went back to his gamekeeping work.

Poppy and Buddy walked over to be with me and both of them put their noses on my shoulders.

'You almost got taken last night,' I said and then promptly burst into tears. I was so grateful that they were still there and I told them how much I loved them. Buddy stared me in the eye for a while and nodded his wise head. I gave him a big kiss on his cheek and he seemed to smile. When he moved away, Poppy rubbed her face on my shoulder, flaring her nostrils and breathing deeply. She stood very still for quite a while just connecting with me. It was the most beautiful moment and it really felt as if they knew what had happened and were grateful that we had helped to keep them safe.

Chapter 18

The time had come to begin our new venture as 'livery yard owners'. Velvet was due to arrive and I was feeling slightly nervous about it.

What if she injures herself in the field? My mind started up it's usual bombardment of worries. *Would Sapna sue us? Why have I agreed to this? It's going to be so much work. I have hardly enough time to do things with Poppy as it is.*

Well it's too late because she's arriving in two hours' time! replied the other side of my brain.

I breathed deeply and tried to relax. I had to take Florence for her riding lesson at Think Like a Pony first and I didn't want her to see me all wound up. We got in the car and Florence chattered excitedly, wondering which pony she would be riding. All I could think about was the impending doom of having to look after somebody else's horse. The weight of the responsibility was so heavy, my chest felt like lead.

Why am I feeling so worried about it? It's only one more horse. It can't be that hard to look after an old horse surely?

I just don't want the responsibility! I don't feel capable of doing this!

But why? I have a horse. It's not like it's anything new. What's wrong with me?

'Mummy! You've missed the turn off!' shouted Florence as we sailed past the lane that led to the riding school. I had been so caught up in my thoughts I had forgotten what I was doing.

'Oh heck! Silly me.' I pulled over so I could turn round. It's never easy turning round on a narrow lane and it all just added to my state of anxiety. Finally, I managed to pull myself together and we arrived just in time for Florence's lesson.

'Hello, Florence!' greeted Mei, one of the instructors, leading a very cute chestnut pony. 'You're going to ride Pumpkin today so it's going to be a bit different.' Florence listened earnestly as Mei took her and Pumpkin into the outdoor school while I leaned over the fence to watch.

'Pumpkin is quite young and he's not done very much so today's lesson is going to be all about you taking responsibility for yourself and him,' continued the instructor. My ears pricked up.

'What do you think I might mean when I say "taking responsibility for yourself"?' asked Mei.

'Er I think it means being aware of what my body is telling him and not being too tense?' asked Florence.

'Yes very good.' Mei smiled. 'Can you think of what else it might mean?'

'Having the confidence to know that I can be a good leader?'

'Excellent.' Mei grinned widely. 'Pumpkin needs to feel your self-confidence and that will help him behave calmly with you. So what can you do to feel and project confidence?'

I couldn't believe what I was hearing. It was such a bizarre coincidence that Florence's lesson was all about feeling confident and taking responsibility. Ever since I had bought Poppy and taken on the field, I felt like I was regularly floundering and unable to cope. I had absolutely no idea where it was coming from and I felt unable to talk about my fears to anyone, even Jack. Maybe it was because I hadn't fully acknowledged my self-doubts until Mei began talking about confidence and responsibility.

'Let's do a self-check before we begin riding,' said Mei. 'Can you wiggle your shoulders?' She continued to go through all the body parts until Florence was wiggling and giggling.

'Excellent, Florence! Definitely no tension anywhere. Now let's see what's going on in your mind. What are you thinking?'

'I'm thinking I can't wait to ride Pumpkin and make him feel really safe,' said Florence. She was standing so confidently, it made me feel very proud.

'Brilliant! Positive thoughts will lead to positive results, so now let's get you on-board.'

Florence led Pumpkin to the mounting block and got on. She was grinning from ear to ear and I noticed that Pumpkin looked very happy and relaxed with her on his back. She walked him round the perimeter of the school in both directions and eventually worked up to trot and canter.

'This is amazing,' said Mei, who had come to stand near me. 'She's the first person to ride Pumpkin in a lesson and her self-confidence is helping him enormously.' I choked up with emotions and found it almost impossible to reply. Luckily, Mei had her full attention on Florence and she went back over to speak with her.

Why can't I feel confident? I wondered. *I'm always worrying about something and feeling that I can't cope. Why? Where is it coming from?*

Florence's lesson finished and interrupted my thoughts which was no bad thing. I pondered on what I had observed all the way to the field where Jack was busy faffing in the school ensuring it was all ready for the arrival of Velvet.

'Ay up, Flo!' she greeted with a wide smile. 'Did you have a good lesson?'

'I rode a new pony called Pumpkin,' Florence replied. 'He looks like Poppy but a lot smaller.'

'That sounds great,' said Jack. 'Oh look out! Here comes trouble!' Toffee ambled over to snuffle around Florence's pockets.

'Let's brush your hair, Toffee. You look very scruffy,' giggled Florence and she led her away which was a relief.

'God, that pony,' said Jack. 'I caught her leaning over the ropes into the school and she pulled out two of the posts. I've just knocked them back in so let's hope it's all ok for Velvet.'

'That sounds like her now,' I said as a roar of an engine approached. I felt my nerves jangling again at the thought of looking after another horse but it was too late now. The horsebox pulled into the carpark and we could hear a lot of neighing coming from inside. Poppy and Buddy looked very interested and came trotting over.

'Oh hell, what to do with these two? We need to get them out of the way before we lead Velvet through to the school,' I panicked. Even though the horses knew each other, it was not a good idea to just let Velvet go straight in the main field with her bad leg in case they all started running around.

'No worries,' said the practical Jack. 'Sapna can drive in and reverse up to the school entrance and she can go straight down the ramp into there.'

Why can't I ever think of these things? I wondered.

Jack went to chat with Sapna while I shooed Poppy and Buddy away from the gate. As the van parked up where Jack directed it, I held my breath for the entrance of Velvet. She certainly was a beauty as she sashayed down the ramp, and although lame on her hind leg she still managed to trot round the school a few times whinnying loudly for all the village to hear.

'Bloody hell! She's got a right voice on her, hasn't she?' laughed

Jack. I was so amazed at how unconcerned and relaxed Jack was about the whole thing. I, on the other hand, was stressed to high heaven with it but I couldn't say anything.

'Yeah she can be very loud,' nodded Sapna.

'Isn't she pretty, Mummy?' said Florence.

'Yes she's very pretty,' I agreed.

Poppy came over first to greet her but Velvet thrust her ears back and bared her teeth as if to say 'Go away!' and Poppy jumped back and came closer to me.

'Oh! That's not very friendly!' I said, giving Poppy a reassuring pat.

'Let's hope she settles down. Might just be because it's all new?' said Jack.

'I hope so.'

Meanwhile, Sapna had driven her horse box back over to the carpark and was unloading an enormous wardrobe of rugs, head collars and several large sacks of feed and a few storage bins. We looked over and watched with open mouths.

'Oh blimey! Where are we going to put all of this?' I asked. 'How many rugs has she got?'

'About a hundred from the looks of it,' grimaced Jack. 'I didn't think about this sort of thing. We'd better see where it can all go.'

'That's everything,' called Sapna. 'I'll leave it with you. See you later!' and without another word or even a goodbye to Velvet, she got back into the driver's seat and started the engine. I opened the gate for her and she drove away.

'That's a bit weird,' said Jack. 'She's just left all this stuff for us to sort out!'

'Yes it's very weird. Bloody hell. We're going to have to fit it all in our feed room.'

The 'feed room' was one of the back rooms in the shelter. It wasn't very big but Jack had the perfect brain with which to create usable space. I watched in awe as she attached ropes along the walls to hang the rugs over and then she fished around under the back section of the shelter (which was slightly raised off the ground) and found some discarded pieces of wood.

'I knew these would come in handy.' She grinned. In no time at all she made some shelves and after shifting all our feed stuff to one side, she managed to get all of Velvet's things into the room.

'Wow!' I said. 'I am amazed!'

'Oh it's nothing.' smiled Jack. 'I was brought up making things so it's second nature now.'

'I wish I could be as practical as you,' I sighed.

'Hmm well, that would take some work!' Jack burst out laughing. 'But seriously, you could do it. After you've watched me for a while, you'll start to see how to do these things.'

'Can we take Toffee out for a walk?' asked Florence. 'She needs to learn self-confidence.'

'A walk?' asked Jack.

'Florence learned all about self-confidence in her lesson today with a new pony,' I explained. 'But I'm not sure whether Toffee is ready to go out yet?'

'Bugger it! Why not?' said Jack. 'We need to do it sometime and maybe Flo can teach us what she learned today?' Florence looked very pleased with herself.

'Do you think this is wise?' I hissed to Jack as Florence went to get Toffee.

'Yeah why not? We won't go far. In fact, why don't you bring Poppy and then me and Flo can follow her with Toffee?'

'That's a good idea. And it gets her away from Velvet, who clearly doesn't like her,' I nodded over to where Velvet was still pulling faces at Poppy. Buddy had wandered off to graze, totally relaxed and unconcerned.

'Right, Flo, are you ready? We're going to bring Pops too. Mum, are you ready?' We were all ready and with some misgivings I set off onto the lane with Poppy, followed by Toffee with Jack and Florence.

'We have to feel confident that we can be a good leader,' I heard Florence explain to Jack. 'And you have to make sure you are relaxed so wiggle your shoulders and that will help.'

'That's great advice,' agreed Jack.

We walked down the lane towards Adam's farm, where there were some young cows in a field. We thought it might be a bit much to take Toffee to see some cows on her first walk out but Florence thought otherwise.

'She needs to learn that we are not afraid of cows, Mummy! Just stand tall and be confident.'

'Ok,' I replied. Jack chuckled.

'Toffee's walking well!' called Jack. 'So keep going!'

Luckily, Poppy wasn't bothered about the cows. She was more interested in eating the grass by their gate and that helped Toffee. But really, Toffee wasn't afraid anyway. She was fascinated by them, especially one that had the same colour pattern as herself. They nosed each other over the wall, which Florence found really funny. It was a great way to relax and stop worrying about Velvet.

'Well I think Toffee has done really well for her first trip out don't you, Flo?' asked Jack.

'Yes. She's a very clever girl aren't you, Toffee?' Florence gave her a hug.

'I think we should go back now and check on Velvet,' I said, worrying that she may have jumped out of the school. Fortunately, all was well when we returned. Velvet was grazing and Buddy was lying down having a snooze nearby. My phone pinged. I assumed it was James so I pulled it out of my pocket to check.

'Oh my God!' My heart felt like it did a forward roll.

'What is it?' asked Jack.

'Read this!' I passed her my phone.

'I saw you just now having a lovely time with that new pony,' Jack read aloud. 'I don't think you're paying enough so I'm doubling your rent from next month.'

'What the hell?' Jack's jaw dropped open.

'Can you believe that?' I was so shocked.

'How can he do that?' Jack was furious. 'I'm going to go and have a word with him!'

'Good luck with that,' I replied. 'He'll tell us to leave!'

'Yes you're right. Hadn't thought of that. God what an awful man!'

I read the text again and didn't know how to respond.

'Don't reply,' said Jack. 'It might make it worse. Just ignore him for now.'

I drove home feeling furious about having the rent doubled especially after I had spent time and money sorting out his ragwort problem, not to mention the fact that we did actually pay our rent unlike the previous woman. But as Jack said, we could do nothing. We had no agreement in writing so we were at the mercy of his peculiarly changeable nature. I couldn't rest though so I messaged Valentina.

'I'm so sorry!' she replied. 'I can't change his mind because he just doesn't care. He will tell you to leave. He isn't bothered if the land is rented or not. I'm so so sorry I tried my best!' I forwarded the conversation to Jack.

'What an arse. Nothing we can do. Twat,' she replied. She was right. There was nothing we could do but it didn't make us feel any better. So on top of the stress of having an extra horse we had extra rent to pay. It was extremely depressing.

Chapter 19

The day spanned before me as clear as a desert. I had nobody booked in for work and Florence was going out with my parents as there was no school for the day. It was so relaxing to take a leisurely shower and not have to do everything at a million miles an hour. Even Wrexford Whippet was lazing around, quite happy to have a snooze on the sofa, and for the first time since we'd got him, he had actually whined to alert us that he needed to go in the garden for a wee. Finally, he had cottoned on to the concept of house-training. Jack and I were going to meet up with Wendy and Gillian for a much-needed fun ride so I was merrily packing a picnic lunch when my phone rang.

'Is that Grace?' asked a man's voice.

'Yes it is. How can I help?' I assumed he wanted to book in for a treatment.

'It's Adam from the farm. I think it's your pony what's got into my bullock field. Ginger and white isn't it?' he asked.

'Oh my God!' I was horrified. 'That's Toffee! How did she get in?'

'Well the little monkey was standin' on that tree stump by the fence and she just seemed to hop over! She's had a good run around with 'em aye!' chuckled Adam. Before I had a chance to reply he had hung up.

Bloody hell! There goes our lovely day out! I could feel my blood pressure rising as I hastily called Jack.

'You'll never guess where Toffee is!' I blurted as soon as she answered.

'Oh no! Where?'

'In Adam's cow field!'

'What? How did she get in there?' Jack sounded as shocked as I was.

'He said she stood on the tree stump and then hopped over!'

'Oh for God's sake. Right, I'll get over there asap!' Jack rang off. Luckily, my parents arrived to take Florence out and they also took Wrexford so I could get straight off to help round up Toffee.

The drive to the field was the opposite of what I had expected it to be like. I had looked forward to a stop off at the shop to get a chocolate milkshake on the way. But instead, I was cursing and fretting and my blood pressure was so high I could have had a heart attack.

What are we going to do with this pony? grumbled my inner voice. *Neither of us has a clue how to train a youngster and she's getting worse by the day! God I can't cope with this, it's just too much!*

Jack arrived at the same time I did and we both parked up and dashed through our fields to get to Adam's cow pasture, which was over the fence, parallel to our back field. Toffee was with the ginger and white bullock that looked like her, peacefully grazing together.

'She looks happy there don't you think? Shall we just leave her?' asked Jack, puffing and panting.

'Wish we could!' I gasped.

'How did she just "hop over" I wonder?' Jack climbed up onto the old oak tree stump and tried to visualise how Toffee had done it without ripping her belly on the barbed wire. 'It just doesn't seem possible.'

'She's very good at doing the impossible,' I replied with a sigh.

'Where's the gate for his field? It's enormous!'

'It must be right over the other side by the road,' I strained to look in the distance to where that field went to. 'We'll have to find out if it's locked. I wonder how safe it is to go in there with all of those young bullocks? Are they likely to come and mob us?'

'I hadn't thought of that, call Adam!'

I rang Adam and luckily, he answered instantly.

'Aye you've got to be careful wi' young beasts. Have you got an umbrella?'

'An umbrella?' I repeated with surprise.

'Aye you know, them things that people use in the rain?' He must have thought I was completely thick.

'Er yes, I know what they are but I haven't got one with me.'

'Well come to my yard and get mine. They don't like umbrellas. If you open and close it at 'em it'll keep 'em away.'

'Ok great! We'll be there in a minute.'

'Umbrella?' asked Jack doubtfully. 'I bloody hope that works. I'll be really annoyed if I get crushed to death by a load of bullocks because of Toffee!'

'Yes it would be a bit inconvenient,' I muttered, silently cursing Toffee. We grabbed her headcollar and a bucket of treats and set off to the farm.

'Now then,' said Adam, handing me an umbrella. 'What you've got to mek sure is that you don't let 'em trample you. These are all very young and inquisitive. They love to play at this age so just watch you don't get crushed, ok?'

'We'll do our best,' I said with a touch of irony.

'Oh crikey,' said Jack when Adam was out of earshot. 'This is a bit hectic!'

'You're telling me! Bang goes our lovely picnic ride.'

Just at that moment, Wendy pulled into the yard and hopped out of her car.

'Hello! What's going on?' she asked.

'Toffee! Toffee is what's going on. I could murder her!' complained Jack.

'Oh no! What's happened?' asked Wendy.

'She's only gone and got into Adam's cow field over there, miles away!' I gestured into the distance where Toffee and the bullocks were having a great time.

'Oh heck! That's a massive field. I'll come and help,' said Wendy and we all set off towards the gate that led into the cow field.

'I can't even see any of them.' I stood on tiptoe, leaning over the gate, scanning the enormous expanse of land that seemed to roll away endlessly.

'I think that's them. They're heading this way!' said Wendy, pointing excitedly.

'Oh thank God for that,' said Jack. 'Right ladies let's go in.' The gate was ancient and held shut with a piece of frayed baler twine so it was a bit fiddly but eventually we managed to get in.

'What shall we do? They seem to be coming quite quickly. Shall we just stand here and wait till they get closer?' I asked.

'Yeah maybe? I've got no idea,' Jack shrugged.

'Yes let's wait and see what they do,' agreed Wendy. 'Look, they're running over now. That's good!' The bullocks had begun to canter and we could see Toffee at the front of the herd, clearly having the best day ever. I was just glad they were heading our way so we could catch her and get on with our ride out.

'They're slowing down now,' I noticed.

'I'll shake the bucket,' said Jack and she began shaking the bucket of treats. The herd sped up again.

'Shit! They're heading straight for us!' said Wendy. The excited bullocks were leaping high in the air, twisting their bodies around in quite a weird and terrifying way.

'Oh my God I'll wave the umbrella!' I squeaked, fumbling to open the huge golf umbrella that Adam had lent us. I pushed the mechanism and slid the umbrella up the shaft and the whole thing fell apart in my hands.

'Bloody hell! Get out now!' yelled Jack and we all dived for the gate.

With a cacophony of moos and the sound of thudding hooves, the entire herd of bullocks barged through the gate, flinging all three of us backwards where we landed in a heap on the ground. We scrambled to get up and to our horror we watched the entire herd run away down the lane with Toffee amongst them.

'Oh no!' we all exclaimed at once.

'What the hell?' came the sound of Adam's voice as he ran out of the yard towards the bedlam. 'Wendy! Call Simon! Tell him to park the tractor across the end of the lane to block 'em. I'll get the quad, you take the Land Rover!' Adam dashed off, leaving Wendy to make the call to the mysterious Simon. Luckily, he answered immediately and as he was in the field at the end of the lane it wasn't a problem for him to block the road.

'God it stinks in here!' I retched as we all climbed into the Land Rover.

'I'm gonna be sick!' said Jack, hastily winding down the windows. Wendy laughed her head off.

'It's vile isn't it?' she guffawed as she drove after Adam, who was speeding down the lane on the quad bike.

'There they are!' I yelled as we rounded a corner and saw the herd of bullocks running away.

'We'll trap them at the end and then drive them back down,' laughed Wendy.

'I don't think we will,' replied Jack as the herd began piling over the half-demolished drystone wall that led onto the golf course.

'Oh. My. God. What the hell do we do now?' I wondered as we watched the bullocks and Toffee leap into the golf course and scatter all over. Terrified golfers abandoned their clubs and ran for safety.

'Bloody hell!' exclaimed Adam as we all jumped out of the smelly Land Rover.

'What shall we do?' asked Wendy. The bullocks were thoroughly enjoying the adventure, trotting around nearby, snorting and sweaty. Most of them began nosing the grass. Toffee got down and rolled.

'We need to be very careful not to scare 'em and make 'em bolt off miles away. Everyone needs to help round the buggers up and drive 'em back over this wall,' said Adam.

Just at that moment, Gillian rode into view on her way to meet us.

'Ah,' she said. 'I see the picnic ride is off and a bit of cow herding is on instead! What tremendous fun!'

'That might not be a bad idea.' Adam nodded. 'It's got their attention.' The bullocks appeared to be very interested in Gillian's horse and came closer to look at her. 'Can you ladies get your horses too? It would be easier to round this lot up.'

'Are you serious?' I couldn't believe my ears. I had never done any cow wrangling and wasn't keen on giving it a go with Poppy.

'Aye I am serious! We'll not get these young 'uns off here easily,' said Adam.

'Right,' said Jack. 'We'll go and saddle up!'

'Be as quick as you can, they're on the move again.' Adam gestured to some of the bullocks who had begun to wander further onto the pristine green. Wendy, Jack and I sped off in the smelly Land Rover to get our horses.

'Why does it stink so bad in here?' I asked, covering my face against the pungent, sickly-sweet aroma. 'I'm literally going to vomit!'

'He had some dead sheep in here yesterday,' chortled Wendy. 'Try not to breathe!'

Fortunately, it wasn't long before we were back at our field and Buddy and Poppy were grazing nearby so we hastily flung tack on and mounted up. They could sense something was going on as they marched out of the gate, ears pricked up.

'Shall we wait for Wendy?' I asked.

'Yeah, good idea,' Jack replied. 'Bloody Toffee! I can't believe this is happening. I hope to God Buddy doesn't freak out when he finds out he has to round up cows!'

'I can't imagine how Poppy is going to react. I hope I don't end up in hospital.' I was feeling nervous.

'You'd better hold on tight, cowboy,' laughed Jack. Before I had time to reply we could hear Denwyn's trotting hooves approaching being led by a jogging Wendy.

'This'll be right up his street,' gasped Wendy, a bit out of breath. 'Denwyn loves the cows!' She scrambled up onto his back.

'Thank God for that,' I said. 'I dread to think what Poppy is going to make of them.'

'Well we'll find out soon,' laughed Wendy.

We trotted up the lane to the golf course where Simon, who turned out to be the weird man in the tractor who almost killed us on our first ride out, was busy dismantling the already semi-demolished drystone wall. His face was completely expressionless.

'Right, ladies you can get in here and aim to drive the buggers back to this spot,' instructed Adam. 'Ride up the edge away from them first and then come round on them.' Wendy led the way and the rest of us followed.

'Oh this is such sport,' trilled Gillian, enthusiastically. 'I've always romanticised about the cowboys out on the range and here we are with this wonderful opportunity to give it a go ourselves!'

'Hmm yes, great,' muttered Jack. 'Bloody Toffee.'

My heart began speeding up and I could feel tension rising. My arms felt heavy and tight.

Oh my God I am going to be sick!

Calm down! insisted the sensible part of my brain.

Calm down? How can I calm down here? Poppy has never done this before. She will be terrified and bolt and I will be thrown off and break my neck and die!

Why should she be afraid of something just because it's new? She might find it interesting and fun? This realisation was like a flash of power. It made me stop and suddenly feel open to a different stream of thought.

I am Mark Rashid, the cowboy. My brain began visualising that I was Mark Rashid, the very experienced horse trainer and cowboy.

I am training all these people how to be a great cowboy like me. I am completely at ease and calm. Poppy knows exactly what to do and she is not bothered at all.

Poppy took a deep breath and lowered her head. I was amazed and relieved. It appeared Poppy had got the measure of the task and she was forward yet relaxed as she strode purposefully onwards and I felt she had read my mind. This helped me to relax even more and see the funny side of the situation.

'Ok ladies!' called Gillian. 'Let's start driving them back! Home! Home on the range!' she began singing. Jack raised her eyebrows and muttered something under her breath.

We turned our horses and began to drive the bullocks forwards. They jumped about a bit and mooed but they began going where we wanted them.

'This is actually quite fun,' I chuckled. 'I certainly wasn't expecting to be doing this ever in my life.'

'Ooh you little monkey! That's my lunch!' shouted Gillian suddenly. Toffee had trotted up alongside and had somehow managed to get her nose into the saddle bag to steal a sandwich, which she gobbled up within seconds. 'That was a beef salad!'

'You have got to be kidding?' Jack was aghast.

'No! She's just eaten some beef, which is a bit ironic isn't it?'

'Bloody Toffee,' sighed Jack for the thousandth time.

'Oh heck!' Wendy called out as a renegade gang of bullocks formed a breakaway group and began trotting in another direction.

'Oh no! What shall we do?' I wailed. I had visions of this going on forever.

'Gillian and Wendy, circle round to your right and go after those buggers. You'll head them off at that bunker with the yellow flag. Me and Grace will keep herding in this direction and then we'll aim to come together down there by that golf cart,' said Jack. Her excellent brain could see exactly what needed to be done.

Why am I so pathetic? I wondered. *Why can't I be as logical and practical as Jack? She never gets in a flap. Why do I always worry about things?*

'Oh for the love of God,' blurted Jack as the greenkeeper suddenly appeared in a mini tractor with a face like thunder.

'What the bloody hell is going on here?' He leaped out of his cab. 'You're ruining my green! Do you have any idea how much work goes into keeping this right?' He yelled, gesticulating wildly with his arms. The bullocks began snorting and prancing around.

'Aaargh!' yelled Wendy as Denwyn reared and snorted.

'Bloody hell!' shouted the man, diving for safety.

Denwyn bucked and Wendy flew off backwards. He neighed ridiculously loudly and bolted for all he was worth into the throng of the bullocks, which set them off running and triggered Gillian's horse to start running too.

'Whoa! Whoa!' I turned Poppy in a tight circle as I could feel her body about to explode. 'You will settle down immediately!' I commanded with a severity I had never heard coming out of my own mouth. Poppy settled and luckily Buddy remained calm too.

'You bloody idiot!' shouted Jack to the man. 'We had it all under control until you came along! Get out of our way and shut the hell up!' The man opened his mouth to retort but thought better of it and backed down.

'Are you ok, Wendy?' I asked as she came hobbling over.

'I think so.' She grimaced. 'What the hell do we do now?'

'Change of tactic,' said Jack. 'We need to get rid of these horses, get the quad bike and lure them all back with a bucket of feed!'

As if on cue, Adam drove up on his quad with a large bucket full of grass nuts.

'I've never in my life seen owt as bloody ridiculous as this,' he said, shaking his head. 'Just shows, doesn't it? Just when you think you've seen it all, summat new happens.' He was remarkably pragmatic about it all. 'You ladies follow behind me and we'll fetch them back with some feed.'

Adam led the way, over the rolling green turf to where we could see the bullocks and the horses in the distance. Fortunately, they had managed to all settle down as they'd run out of steam so they didn't bother to react when we got close by.

'There's nothing like a good gallop to blow the cobwebs away,' greeted the irrepressible Gillian with a cheery wave.

'Right ladies, you keep back over there and I'll shake this bucket,' instructed Adam.

We all hung back and the bullocks responded like magic to the sound of the feed being shaken. Like the pied piper, Adam began driving, followed by the entire herd of bullocks, Toffee and Denwyn and we riders brought up the rear.

In no time at all we were back through the by now completely dismantled drystone wall and back onto the lane. With the tractor driving behind us all we managed to get the bullocks back into their field and catch Toffee and Denwyn.

'What a marvellous day,' laughed Gillian in her sing-song voice. 'It's one for the diary, isn't it?'

'I need a stiff drink now. Bloody Toffee! What the hell am I going to do with you?' Jack pulled a face.

Toffee was thoroughly exhausted from the escapade so we took her home and made her a big feed. Jack checked her all over and luckily there were no injuries.

'Seriously though,' said Jack, 'what are we going to do about

Toffee? I really regret buying her.'

'Could you sell her?' I wondered aloud.

'Hmm. I know I should but even though she's bloody annoying I would only want her to go to a good home,' replied Jack. 'I suppose it was always the plan to sell her but I wanted to train her first. Realistically it's a bit too much work isn't it?'

'Yes and it's work we don't really know how to do.'

'Yeah,' sighed Jack. 'Ok, can you help write the ad?'

'Yes. I'll have a go tonight.' I nodded.

I drove home full of mixed emotions. On the one hand I felt relieved to think Toffee could be leaving soon but on the other I felt sad because I cared about her and it wasn't her fault that we were too ignorant to know how to manage her. The thought of her being sold to a stranger filled me with dread. Also, I knew that Florence would be devastated. She loved Toffee and had a special connection with her.

My mind suddenly moved onto the memories of the mad day we had. The thing that struck me the most was how I had managed to stop Poppy from bolting after the others. It felt like an enormous achievement and I smiled as I realised how capable I could be. It really hit home how much the thoughts I chose to think affected not only my emotions and how my body worked but also Poppy and her reactions. I became very aware that I needed to learn even more about that aspect of horsemanship, but how and where? I was learning a lot by watching Florence in her riding lessons but I wished I could have my own lessons too.

Chapter 20

I looked out of my window to check the weather before I headed out to the field. It was that really annoying temperature where it's not exactly cold but it's not warm either. I sighed and stuffed some extra clothes into a bag just in case I needed another layer, then I dashed out of the house before I could see the laundry mountain and feel guilty about it. I wanted to do a bit of horsemanship with Poppy to see how deep a connection we could have, even though I didn't know how or what I was going to do in order to achieve it.

Who the hell is that woman leaning over our gate? I wondered as I pulled into the layby. *Oh it's Sapna!*

'Hello!' I called out to her. 'Are you ok?'

'I can't get in! I don't know the gate code.'

'Oh right! I'll open it, hang on a mo.' I was surprised she hadn't bothered to ask us what the code was when she brought Velvet, and even more surprised that she hadn't been to see her until now. I opened the gate and Sapna went in to see her horse while I brought my car in.

Velvet was very pleased to see her owner and dashed to the rope-fence to greet her.

'Ahh is she still all alone in here? I thought you might have let her out by now.'

'We wanted to make sure everyone was settled first because she's been a bit aggressive towards Poppy.'

'Well I think she's had long enough. She's an old girl so I'm sure it'll be fine now if she goes out,' said Sapna, and before I could reply, she opened the gate and let Velvet out of the school and into the main field. Velvet snorted and trotted off at top speed despite her limp.

'Ha! She's full of it!'

'Yes,' I didn't know what else to say as I was a bit apprehensive.

'You see it's all ok,' said Sapna smiling. 'Oh shit!' The smile faded into a frown as Velvet kicked out at Poppy's hind leg and then she spun around as quick as a ninja and bit her bottom. 'Oh God! Velvet!' she yelled. 'She's never done that before.' Sapna and I both ran over to where Poppy was standing, stunned and bleeding.

'Not again! She's always the one who gets injured.' I was extremely annoyed.

'I'm so sorry! I'm actually a vet nurse so I'll sort it.' Sapna dashed to her car and came back with a first aid box. It was a superficial wound so it didn't take much to clean it up but Poppy was lame so that was the end of my horsemanship plan.

'It's just a bit swollen so the lameness should wear off in a day or so,' said Sapna, handing me a few sachets of bute. 'Give her one a day for three days. I'll take Velvet for a walk around the fields.'

I was fuming and texted Jack to tell her what had happened.

'Silly cow!' she replied. 'I'll come up later and check on Poppy. I'm just in the middle of a job.' I sighed and stood with Poppy, who looked upset.

'Poor Poppy. It's always you who gets injured isn't it?' Poppy seemed to nod as if in agreement. I sighed again and decided to clear some of the endless poos that the horses kindly produced for us almost constantly.

'You're always shovelling shits,' laughed a familiar voice at my shoulder, sending me into orbit.

'Christ! You nearly gave me a heart attack!'

'I'm a hunter,' chuckled Rob. 'You'll never catch me sneaking up on you.'

'You're annoying, I know that much.' I didn't know whether to laugh or tell him off.

'What are you up to now? Apart from shit shovelling of course,' he asked.

'Nothing now that my horse is lame. Why?'

'I could do with some help if you're up for it.' Rob pursed his already thin lips and narrowed his icy blue eyes.

'Er, maybe?' I replied cautiously. 'Tell me more.'

'The geese are all on the wrong field and I need you to help me move them. I can't be spotted doing it cos I'll lose my job so I need you to be my driver.'

'Why do you need to move them? And how do you move a load of geese?' It was such an absurd request.

'Right, good questions. The thing is, we've managed to get an out of season licence to shoot the geese and I've got a party of Saudi princes booked in for a shoot tomorrow, but the geese have been on a field that belongs to the estate at Rington all week. I'm not allowed to shoot on that field so I want to scare them off so they go to feed on one of our fields instead. At least that's the plan anyway. I can't let the earl know I'm doing this though because it's not really the done thing.'

'This all sounds a bit bonkers to me. What do you need me to actually do?' I asked.

'Just drive me over to that field and then drive me away again.' Rob smiled.

'Sounds easy enough.' I nodded. 'Ok let's go!' I put my barrow away and we walked over to my car.

'I'll park at the pub. Get me from there,' said Rob as he got into his pickup. It didn't take long to get to the pub and Rob got into my car carrying an olive duffel bag.

'Just drive down this road and then take the first left,' he directed, pushing the passenger seat as far back as it would go to accommodate his ridiculously long legs.

The turnoff was a single lane dirt track that wound past a beautiful yet decrepit farm and overgrown fields. Rabbits hurried in all directions to escape the car and I slowed down so that I didn't squash any.

'Ok, you can park up anywhere here,' said Rob eventually, scraping his wavy, toffee-coloured hair into a little bun at the back of his head.

'Wow!' I said as I stepped out of the car. We had come to an enormous field which was teeming with geese. There must have been thousands of them. I'd never seen or heard anything like it in my life. They were all honking away to each other so noisily, like a load of football fans at a big match. I leaned over the gate and tried to count them but it was impossible.

'It's a sight to behold, isn't it?' replied Rob as he jumped out of the car. 'All the geese in the neighbourhood are right here. But not for long.'

'Why are you shooting them, the poor things?'

'People always ask us why. Can you see the damage they're doing to this barley field? If we don't cull them, there'll be no crops.'

'Oh right, yes. It's still so sad though, isn't it?'

'It is sad, yes. Geese mate for life and if one of them dies the other will often mourn for the rest of its life.'

'Oh no! That's awful! How can you shoot them?'

'Well, we do our best to get the pairs. They often graze together and they'll be the same size as each other usually too. So like look over there. Can you see the smaller pair there and then the larger pair next to them? They choose partners that are similar so it helps us to get both of them.'

'Oh well, that's some consolation I suppose.' My heart felt very heavy looking at the beautiful birds who were enjoying themselves eating barley and chatting with their friends.

'When I was learning about shooting as a lad, there weren't that many geese here but the population has grown so much they're completely decimating the crops. If people hadn't murdered nearly all the big birds of prey years ago there'd be a better balance of nature. But they did so now it's down to people like me to make sure they don't eat all our food.'

He pulled a pair of binoculars out of his pocket and looked around to check there was no one around. 'Great, it's all clear.'

'How are you going to move them?' I asked.

'With these,' Rob grinned and opened his duffel bag. He checked once more that no one was around and then pulled out two large fireworks.

'You can't be serious?'

'I'm always serious! Here you grab one.' He thrust a rocket into my hand.

'What? No way!' I thought he was joking.

'It's fine! We just need to hold them above our heads and let them go.' Before I could reply, Rob pulled a lighter out of his pocket and lit the rockets. 'Hold it high!' he commanded and stunned with shock, I dumbly held the rocket as high as I could.

With a fizz, the rockets shot in the air exploding loudly over the field. The geese let out a mass roar of shrieks as they hurtled into the air to fly for their lives. The sound was deafening as a million wings beat in fury.

'Get back in the car!' shouted Rob and we both dashed back to the car and dived in. 'Quick! Drive before anyone sees us!'

'Where to?' I yelled.

'The pub!'

I shot off down the winding lane at top speed, my heart racing. We got to the pub in seconds and I parked in the furthest corner of the carpark.

'Oh my God! I can't believe we just did that!'

'I know! Fun wasn't it?' laughed Rob. He pulled his phone out of his pocket. 'Three, two, one ...' His phone began ringing.

'Now then?' said Rob winking at me and putting his phone on speaker so I could listen in.

'Now then,' replied a deep and rather old sounding voice. 'Did you hear them explosions just now?'

'No. I'm in the pub having some food. What explosions?'

'Well, I was just up on top bank on the quad, you know, and there were two really loud bangs like proper explosives.'

'Oh right? No I didn't hear it. I'm in the pub, mate,' said Rob biting his lip trying not to laugh.

'Hmm. Well I don't know,' I could almost hear the man scratching his head with confusion. 'All them geese have buggered off now and I needed 'em on there for a shoot at weekend, you know.'

'Oh nightmare. Well I can't help you, mate. Like I said I'm just at the pub with a friend,' Rob smirked.

'Oh right. Ok feller. If you find out owt about it let me know,' said the crestfallen man.

'Yeah will do, mate.' Rob hung up and promptly burst out laughing. 'Oh my God!' he guffawed, tears streaming down his rough cheeks. 'He'll be shitting it now!'

'Who was that?' I asked laughing at Rob's infectious laughter.

'He's the Rington gamekeeper and he's been boasting all week about the geese on that field! Ah he's not boasting any more, is he?' Rob shook with laughter. 'Those geese won't be back there in a hurry!'

'They'll never go there again,' I laughed deep from my belly. The kind of laughter I hadn't experienced since being at school when life was simple and there were no responsibilities. It felt so liberating to have done something so hilarious and naughty.

'Right, I suppose I'd better get back to work,' said Rob eventually with a sigh. 'Thanks for helping. We'll go on another adventure soon if you like?'

'Yes definitely! That was so funny.' Rob stepped out of my car and waved. I sighed deeply and drove back to the field to see how Poppy was doing. I felt a wave of annoyance wash over me as I remembered her new injury. I could do without extra stress, especially after having had such a good laugh.

Sapna had gone by the time I got back and despite the bute, Poppy was hobbling around still looking sorry for herself. I stood in the field observing her for a while unsure of what to do.

'Oh dear! What happened to Poppy?' called a voice behind me. It was Gillian, leaning over the gate. She was wearing what appeared to be a 1970's style kaftan in peacock blue with orange and silver embroidery. It was beautiful but completely incongruent with her farming lifestyle.

'She got kicked by Velvet earlier,' I grumbled, walking over to the gate.

'Do you need any bute?' asked Gillian kindly.

'She's just had one but it doesn't seem to be doing much yet,' I replied.

'Hmm. Well, if it doesn't wear off in a day or so I'd be inclined to call Marcus. He's marvellous at fixing injured horses.'

'Who's Marcus? Is he a physio?'

'Not a physio as such but he's a very gifted horseman and healer. A rare specimen in this day and age. He does Neurostructural Integration Technique. Have you heard of it?'

'No. It sounds interesting.'

'It's marvellous! I'll give you his number.' Gillian fished around in her apparently endless pocket and eventually found her phone and gave me his number. Bizarrely, I felt inexplicably drawn to making an appointment so when Gillian went on her way, I texted him immediately.

'Hi I got your number from Gillian and I was just wondering if you could see my horse, Poppy?'

'Yes I should be able to. Where are you?' came his immediate response, which I wasn't expecting. I replied with my address.

'I'm in your area tomorrow late morning and I've just had a cancellation if you want a visit?' text Marcus.

'Wow! Yes please!' I replied eagerly and then texted him the directions.

Why have I booked an appointment for some weird treatment with a man I don't know? I suddenly felt annoyed with myself. *I didn't even ask how much it costs. James will go mad.*

Don't tell him! said the sneaky part of my brain.

How can I not tell him? He'll find out when I pay for it. Damn. Why didn't I just wait and see how she is in a few days? He's bound to be a nutter if Gillian knows him. He didn't even ask what's wrong with her. God what have I done?

For some unknown reason, it didn't occur to me to call him and cancel so I drove home, chuntering to myself almost endlessly about how much it might cost and wondering if it would even work.

Chapter 21

I awoke to the sound of the dog whining so I leaped out of bed.

Why does nobody else bother to let the dog out in the morning? I was stressed about the forthcoming visit from Marcus and didn't want to have to begin the day with wee and poo everywhere.

There was wee and a poo right near the door. Unfortunately, it was near the door I had to open inwards – into the kitchen – so it made a large smelly smear across the tiles and of course it got right into the grout edges which took ages to clean properly. What a way to start the day.

'Oh Wrexford! You stinky boy!' laughed Florence when she came in for her breakfast.

'Why are you wearing a swimming costume?' I asked in horror. 'Look at the time! You need to get your uniform on!'

'But we are starting swimming lessons today, Mummy,' replied Florence very matter-of-factly.

'Yes but that doesn't mean you need to wear a swimming costume now! You need to go and get your uniform on!' I gasped.

'Are we swimming in our uniforms?' Florence looked very confused and it took several minutes to explain that she would be changing when she got there. She insisted on wearing her costume under her uniform and by that time I just couldn't be bothered to argue.

'Let's just get in the car and you can have a jam sandwich for breakfast on the way.' I had given up on the battle of healthy breakfasts a while ago. I felt so guilty letting her eat jam and white bread for breakfast, knowing how many other little princesses would be eating porridge and fruit or eggs and wholemeal toast.

So long as she eats something that's all that matters surely? I hoped that was the case.

As usual, it was impossible to park anywhere near school and I felt very sorry for all the local residents who had to put up with the terrible parking every morning. One man was swearing his head off about a car that was blocking him in his drive and he used a four-letter word beginning with c, which of course Florence overheard and wanted to know what it meant.

'It's not a word that nice people say. Oh look at that cute dog!' I tried to change the subject.

'Yes but what does it mean, Mummy?' Florence was not letting it go.

'I don't know, Florence.'

'Ok well I will ask my teacher and then I'll let you know what it means.' And with that she ran off ahead to one of the girls in her class who was just walking in to school.

'Jasmine!' shouted Florence. 'Does your mummy know what c*** means?' I was rooted to the spot, open mouthed in shock, as was the mother of said child. She was a particularly snooty mother who I had never spoken to and never wanted to speak to. She looked at me with such disgust that all I could do was shrug my shoulders and pull a face. I turned and walked back to the, car stifling the urge to roar with laughter, but fortunately I remembered to quickly phone the school to explain why Florence might be using that word.

Wrexford was walked at break-neck speed which suited him down to the ground and then I dashed home to treat the only person I had booked in for the morning. Work completed, I then gorged on a large slice of chocolate cake while simultaneously stuffing a mountain of laundry into the washing machine, changed into my field clothes and leaped into the car.

Aaaand breathe! said the yoga-teacher section of my brain.

I took a deep breath and arrived at the field slightly less frazzled than I had been all morning. Poppy was still lame so I gave her another bute which seemed to work fairly quickly, and I noticed that Toffee was not doing anything naughty which was a relief. It was very calm and peaceful up at the field and it was very relaxing to observe the little pied wagtails, bobbing around pecking at the ground, looking for worms. Summer had arrived and the dandelions were popping up all over the field like fluffy yellow pompoms along with velvety clumps of red clover, which the horses loved. The distant hum of a tractor added to the wonderful sensation of being in the countryside and my heart felt very happy. I gave Poppy a groom to make sure she looked her best before Marcus arrived and just as I'd finished brushing her lustrous ginger tail, his car pulled into the carpark.

I don't know about you, but I always create an image in my mind before I meet someone and I had visualised Marcus to be of medium height, slim with blond curly hair. I could not have been more wrong. He opened his car door and swivelled around, unfolding his extremely long, spindly legs before stepping out and stretching. The buttons on his smart tweed waistcoat were strained to the limit and looked like they might burst due to his enormously rotund girth. But the feature that struck me the most was his waxed, black curly moustache which was reminiscent of Hercule Poirot. It was really hard to not stare at it.

'Hello! I'm Marcus. Are you Grace?' he greeted cheerily in a lovely Durham accent.

'Hi, yes!'

Stop looking at his moustache! barked my inner parent.

I can't help it! Why has he got a moustache like that?

'Is this Poppy then?' asked Marcus, striding over to her. Poppy gave him a sniff and seemed to approve of him.

'Yes,' I replied giving her a little scratch.

God. Why have I booked this? He's clearly a total weirdo with that moustache. And why are his eyes so green? They must be contact lenses. Nobody has eyes that colour. I bet this is going to be the biggest waste of money and James is going to go nuts.

'Ok well how I usually start is I ask the owner to lead the horse around in both directions so I can see what's going on. So can you just walk her over to that hedge and back?' asked Marcus. I nodded and began leading Poppy over to the other side of the field.

He still hasn't asked what's wrong with her and he's not going to see anything now that the bute has worked. What a waste of time, I chuntered inwardly. Poppy walked perfectly over to the hedge and back.

'Right, that's fine. Bring her into the car park and I'll treat her in here away from the other horses,' said Marcus opening the gate for me to lead her through.

'So I can see she's lame on that leg,' said Marcus pointing to the exact leg. 'Probably from one of the others kicking her I reckon. And it's knocked her off balance right up her spinal line to her head which is why she carries it slightly to the side to try to rebalance.'

'Does she?' I hadn't noticed.

'Yes, I'll show you.' Marcus led her back into the field and walked her. Despite not displaying any signs of lameness, she was holding her head to one side in a very odd way.

'How did you know she was lame?' I asked, intrigued.

'I can feel it.' Marcus smiled. 'She also doesn't like her right side being groomed because she's got a tiny impingement on a superficial nerve, but we'll get that sorted.'

I was stunned. Poppy had reacted to being groomed on her right side ever since I had started with her and I was still to find a brush that didn't annoy her.

'How did you know that?' I couldn't believe it.

'She just told me,' Marcus replied with a shy sort of smile and I was too shocked to say anything.

I stood open mouthed as he began his work. It was a peculiar sort of technique involving small manipulations followed by moments of rest. It looked very methodical.

'Can I ask, what you're actually doing?' It looked so odd.

'Of course you can ask. So what I'm doing is creating a conversation on a physical level. It's a multi-faceted, systematic approach to help the horse correct itself. I'm generating reflex and that corrects the musculo-skeletal structure as well as vibration on a frequency level which helps the cranial sacral connection. The aim is to rebalance by connecting the brain to the body. Similar to what a chiropractor or osteopath is trying to achieve but on more levels.'

'Wow,' I replied. My brain felt like it was swimming in treacle trying to understand what he had just said. Eventually I had to admit defeat and accept I had absolutely no idea.

'How did you hear her telling you about not liking to be groomed?' I was fascinated by that.

'I don't really know,' said Marcus thoughtfully. 'I've always been able to hear them speak. Poppy is a particularly chatty horse.'

'Is she? How funny! What's it like? How do you hear it?'

'Well now hmm. That's a tough question. I think I've been blessed with a gift from my grandad. He was a proper Gypsy horseman. It's hard to describe. I feel it and I hear it and also they send me pictures. It's like they'll pick something they think will be familiar to me. I think they have a photographic album in their brain so they match a picture that they feel I'll get or they use a voice that they think I'll understand.'

'Wow that's so bizarre. My brain is completely boggled by that! Is she saying anything else?'

'Yes,' he nodded. 'She says she really misses the old yard because she enjoyed going into the arena and doing schooling with you.'

'No way,' I was gobsmacked. 'We did do a lot of schooling! How did you know I wasn't always here?'

'She just told me,' laughed Marcus. 'She also said you need to work on your balance because when she canters you always end up on her neck.'

'No way? I do! And I don't know why!'

'You might just need to work on your core strength,' suggested Marcus. 'Maybe a bit of Pilates?'

I pondered on his words as he continued his manipulations on Poppy. She looked like she was thoroughly enjoying it and yawned widely as she released a load of tension.

'She's saying you need to relax more because you're always

turning up feeling stressed about something,' said Marcus after a while.

'That's true.' I grimaced, remembering my hectic morning and wishing I could put in place everything I'd learned in Wales. 'It's not easy to remember to relax though is it?'

'Yes it does take a lot of work. We need to always make an effort to practise.'

'I'd love to know about her first home,' I said. 'Can you ask her where she came from?' Poppy shot me a look that sent a chill down my spine. Her ears flattened against her head and her eyes narrowed. It looked for all the world as if she had understood what I had said.

'Oh dear,' said Marcus. 'It wasn't nice.'

'What is she saying?' I began to feel my heart thumping in my chest.

'Well, she said there were two girls who used to beat her and make her run very fast. She didn't like them. And she misses her mum. She doesn't know why she was tied to a post while they led her mum away. She was left tied to the post for days until she stopped struggling.' Marcus's eyes filled with tears and he coughed and focussed on his work again. 'She said she learned how to do as she was told so that they'd stop hitting her.'

My mouth dropped open with silent shock and I felt sick to the stomach.

'That's awful!' I said when I finally felt able to speak. I remembered how robotic she was when I first tried lunging her and then I remembered her fearful reaction to the whip.

'Yes it's disgusting. But sadly, it's not uncommon.'

We were silent for a while and then I gave Poppy a hug and she relaxed and yawned again.

'She's a happy girl now though.' Marcus smiled. 'She says she loves being with you.'

'I love being with her,' I choked back the tears and gave her another hug.

'Right, we're all done,' said Marcus eventually. I couldn't believe an hour had already passed by. 'Let her rest for a couple of days and then just take her out for a walk in-hand before riding again. She'll need a a follow-up visit in a fortnight.'

I felt a bit of a zombie after Marcus drove away. It was as if he had released something in me too but I couldn't put my finger on what.

A following day I was catching up with admin work when my phone rang. I was surprised to see it was Bernie, Poppy's previous owner.

'You'll never guess what's just happened!' she shouted, I had to hold the phone away from my ear to avoid being deafened. 'I'm bloody fuming!'

'What's happened?'

'I've just been to get some new tyres on my car and you won't bloody believe this!' she was enraged and I didn't understand why she was calling me to tell me about her car, which I assumed was the problem.

'Er right?' I replied. 'What happened?'

'The guy who did the tyres is a family friend and he said, "You see that feller over there? He's the man who sold Poppy to your brother. He's a right git I don't know why he's come in here after what he did to that poor horse." And I said what do you mean so he said he used to let these two young lasses beat the crap out of her so that she'd learn to do as she's told! So that's why our Dave bought her to rescue her and I just thought he was mad to buy a big horse for my little girl!' Bernie burst into tears. I was shocked into total silence.

'All these years and I had no idea about any of that!' she cried. 'Well, I went over to him and I told him what I thought of him and can you bloody believe it? He said nothing and just walked away. He said nothing! I wanted to thump him but I stopped myself. Don't know how but I did!'

'Thank God for that,' I said. 'He isn't worth getting into trouble with the police. What a vile and horrible man!'

'I'm so glad our Poppy's found you and now she's loved,' sighed Bernie before she had to dash off.

'Bloody hell!' I said out loud to myself as her words sank in. 'That's what Marcus said! Two girls beating her!' I was completely stunned. How did he know? I was dying to know more about Marcus and his peculiar gift of being able to hear horses speak and could hardly wait to see him again.

Chapter 22

'Shouldn't you be riding him?' The man cocked his head as if to emphasise the fact that it was really weird for me to be walking my horse down the lane. I didn't know his name. He was one of the regular walkers and he always seemed to be wearing a pair of shorts even if it was raining.

'Not today! She's just getting over an injury,' I replied.

'Oh poor lad. He's a handsome horse isn't he?' The man patted Poppy's neck.

'Yes. She's very beautiful!' I nodded.

'Well I hope he gets better soon!' and the man went on his way.

How bizarre! I mused to myself and continued walking.

It was a very pleasant experience to walk with Poppy. It felt strangely relaxing and I noticed a rhythm between us. Not just our footsteps but also our breathing. Every now and again we stopped to enjoy the terrific scenery.

'Aren't we lucky to be here?' I sighed. Poppy breathed deeply, flaring her nostrils, picking up a scent of something. 'It's just so beautiful. Look at the water, it's shimmering like a mirror.' The reservoir could be seen through the pine trees and looked like a glorious lake. We walked on past lush, green meadows dotted with black and white cows and golden barley fields that wafted in the breeze and all around, birds were singing and butterflies were flitting about trying to find a mate.

'Oh wow a stoat!' I exclaimed as a long, brown furry little thing dashed across the lane and then dived into a hole in the drystone wall.

We walked for quite some time and it dawned on me that I had taken her to places I wouldn't feel confident if I had been riding. Places I assumed would make her jumpy for various reasons, all of which were probably in my head. Poppy was so relaxed and visibly enjoying exploring. I was relaxed because I didn't fear 'falling off if she spooks and bolts' and I remembered that walking in-hand was one of the things that Elise, my riding instructor, and Jim, the traveller, had suggested I do more of. I hadn't made the time to do it because I prioritised riding, believing that to be more valuable. But I suddenly realised the depth of importance of simply walking with a horse. I felt so wonderfully calm and I loved being able to talk to her and see her facial expressions.

'I suppose we'd better head back for home,' I remarked, glancing at my watch. 'We've had a lovely time, haven't we?' We ambled leisurely back to the field and as I turned her loose, she stopped to give me a little nuzzle on my shoulder. It felt like that was her way of saying, 'Thank you I enjoyed that.'

Velvet wandered over and nickered at me. I was surprised because she'd been quite aloof and I hadn't wanted to interact with her after her being so mean to Poppy. But there she was asking for some attention and her eyes looked so soft I couldn't be cross with her any more.

'Hello, Velvet,' I greeted. She rubbed her head on my chest so I gave her a scratch. 'I need to get on with some shit shovelling now.' I walked off to get the barrow and Velvet walked with me. She stayed with me the entire time and it felt surprisingly lovely. We chatted about the birds, the multitude of weeds and other things I could see nearby. Even though it was just me talking to her, it felt like a two-way conversation. Velvet seemed quite wise and I would have loved to have been able to hear what she might have been saying back to me.

The poo clearing done, I sat down on the mounting block to eat a sandwich (I did wash my hands first). Even though I hadn't ridden, I felt the same sensation of fulfilment that I often had after a ride. It dawned on me how special it was to just *be* with a horse and enjoy whatever it was about them that made them so enchanting.

'Bloody hell! This gate is really annoying!' I jumped at the intrusion. It was Sapna, almost fighting with the slider on the gate. It was very awkward and needed to be refitted but that was Jack's department.

'Oh yes, sorry it needs fixing,' I replied.

'Well do you think you can bloody well get on and do it? I'm paying good money to keep my horse here and I don't expect to have to battle with the gate to get in!' Sapna's face twisted up with rage as she stormed past me into the field shelter. I was completely taken aback by the force of her aggression. I felt shaky as if I'd been smacked in the face and my hands became suddenly very weak. It was horrible. I didn't know what to do so as I had finished everything I needed to do, I got in my car and left.

Should I have said something? Why didn't I say anything?
I was shocked! What could I have said?
God that was awful!

My mind went round and round like a terrible roundabout, repeating itself endlessly about what I could have said but didn't. Eventually, life chores took my attention and I forgot all about it. By the end of the day I managed to brush it aside and put it down to Sapna probably just having a bad day.

The following day, Jack and I had arranged to meet for a ride. I arrived at the field to find her dismantling the gate slider.

'Oh I'm glad you're fixing that. Sapna was furious about it yesterday,' I said.

'Well it's sorted now,' grinned Jack. 'What a silly thing to be furious about. Right, where's my horse?' Jack walked off whistling a merry tune and I called Poppy over. Miraculously she actually came over looking very enthusiastic, which I felt was a result of our lovely walk yesterday.

We tied the horses to the car park fence and groomed in the sun, chatting about where we could explore. There were so many new rides to try.

'Have you fixed the gate yet?' Sapna had suddenly appeared by the gate.

'Yes it's working fine now,' Jack replied, smiling. 'How are you settling in?'

'I want to drive my car in so can you move your horses out of the bloody way? I'm sick of parking on the road and I don't see why I should when I'm paying you so much.' Sapna stomped off to her car.

'What the hell?' Jack was as shocked as I was. 'What's got into her?'

'She was like that yesterday,' I replied. I felt glad that Jack was with me. We moved the horses and Sapna drove in. Without a word of thanks, she strode off towards the shelter. Jack raised her eyebrows and looked at me quizzically.

'I'll go and speak to her,' I whispered and walked after Sapna. She was in the field shelter, rummaging in the feed room and muttering to herself.

'Hi Sapna. Are you ok? Has something upset you?'

Sapna turned to face me. 'Why don't you mind your own fucking business?' and with that she turned away and continued doing whatever it was she'd been doing.

I felt like I'd been punched in the stomach as I walked back to Jack with jelly legs.

'Let's tack up and get out of here,' I gasped, holding back the desire to cry. I didn't want to look pathetic in front of Jack. We tacked up, hastily mounted and trotted out of the gate.

'What happened?' asked Jack when we were out of hearing range.

'All I said was "Are you ok? Has something upset you?" and she told me to "Mind my own fucking business" really aggressively! So I just walked away. I'm shocked!'

'Do you think she's got a problem in her personal life?'

'Maybe? But even so, it's not the way to speak to someone is it?' I shuddered at the memory.

'No, you're right, it isn't.' Jack shook her head. 'Who would speak like that at our age? Maybe when you're like fifteen or something but not now.'

'Yes that's true.' My mind went back to school days. 'It was a bit like a teenage sort of interaction. I wish I'd said something back to her now. I don't know why I didn't. I was so shocked.'

'You know there was this girl in my year at school who used to be a right cow and I was absolutely terrified of her.' Jack frowned at the memory. 'I never dared to stand up to her. Wish I had!'

'Really? I'm surprised. I can't imagine you being afraid of anyone.'

'Well looks can be deceiving,' she sighed. 'I can't believe how bloody rude Sapna was! I'm gonna say something to her later when she's calmed down.'

We rode on in silence for a while, enjoying the calming sensation of being surrounded by beautiful countryside. After a while, all thoughts of Sapna had left our minds and Jack told me about her plans to dig out the stream at the bottom of the field to make it more of a drinking hole for the horses.

'So I don't think it'll be too big a job,' she concluded as we rode back into the carpark and dismounted.

'You need to do something about that bloody pony!' snarled Sapna as she marched through the field gate into the carpark. 'It's taken ages to groom Velvet because Toffee kept getting in the way! I had to give her a kick in the chest eventually.'

'You did what?' sputtered Jack.

'I kicked her. It's only what another horse would do. She needs to learn some manners and you two are obviously not teaching her anything except how to be annoying,' declared Sapna eyeing Jack with such power I could see her wilting. 'Anyway, I'm going now.' And with that she got into her car, slammed the door and drove away. Jack sat down on the mounting block, her mouth open in shock.

'Oh my God!' she stuttered. 'She's awful!'

'I had no idea what a total bitch she was,' I replied with a shaky voice. 'What are we going to do? We need to get rid of her!'

'We do, but how? I don't want to speak to her again and we do need her money now that Roger's doubled the rent.'

'Oh hell yes the rent. We'll just have to advertise and find someone else.'

'What if we end up with someone even worse than her? If someone who seemed nice can become so vile what the hell would a total stranger be like? Let's give it a couple of weeks and see if she calms down.' Jack mopped her brow and breathed deeply.

'Ok,' I agreed. 'I'd better get going so I'll see you later.'

As I drove towards the shops my mind went back to my school days. It had begun when I was about nine in a quiet sort of a way that creeps up on you without you noticing. Little events such as stealing my pencil case for a laugh morphed into her whispering to other girls while looking over at me and then they would giggle. I don't know why my automatic reaction was to try to appease her and make her be my friend. She was never my friend. I would wake up every morning with a heavy sensation of dread bubbling around in my stomach and during the drive to school my heartrate would speed up.

Sometimes she would be really lovely and would sit next to me in class and suggest fun games to play at break time. Then the following day she would tease me by hiding things or laugh at my shoes or whisper. It was the whispering that got to me the most. The other girls would all laugh and would never tell me what it was about. I would feel hot and my cheeks would go red while nausea would rise into my tight and choked up throat. I would fight to keep back the tears. What a total bitch she was.

But I'm an adult now. I don't have to put up with Sapna's behaviour, I reasoned.

She's so aggressive, though. I don't know what to say to her. I hope she doesn't come up every day. Why isn't she at work?

My mind cycled round and round until at last it was school pickup time and all my attention got swallowed up.

'Can we go and see Toffee?' asked Florence as she danced out of the school playground. I glanced at my watch.

'Yes, I suppose so for a quick visit.'

As we approached the field, I noticed my heart rate had increased and I felt anxious.

I hope Sapna isn't there. I can do without seeing her again.

I breathed a sigh of relief when I saw the gate was locked and no one was there.

'Toffee!' called Florence as she jumped out of the car. 'Where are you?'

'Probably in the shelter.' I hoped. 'Let's go and see!'

Toffee was not in the shelter. I scanned the field. Nothing. My heart sank.

'Oh heck! Where can she be?' I wondered out loud. 'We'd better go to the bottom of the field and check down there.' Florence sprinted ahead and I trotted to keep up, my mind whirring with all the terrible possibilities of what Toffee might be doing.

'Oh for God's sake, Toffee!' I shouted. 'How have you got through there?' Toffee had managed to get half of her body through the ancient stock fencing at the very bottom of the field. She wasn't remotely concerned that the back half of her body was still in our field as she munched happily on the wheat growing in the neighbouring field.

'Toffee! You naughty girl!' Florence chided. 'Get back in here immediately!' But Toffee couldn't go backwards or forwards. She was stuck.

'Oh for God's sake!' I blazed. 'You are so annoying, Toffee!' Just at that moment, Simon, the grumpy farmer who hated horse riders, trundled into the field in his tractor. 'That's all we need.'

He looked over at us, his eyes narrowed and his mouth curled into huge irritation.

'Damn,' I sighed as he jumped out of his tractor and strode towards us.

'Grrsnff,' he grumbled. 'It's bloody stuck isn't it? Bloody 'ell.' He muttered some more incoherent words and stomped back towards his tractor. I didn't know what to say or do. He leaned into the cab, grabbed something and stalked back over.

'Geeyaa, harumph,' mumbled Simon and he brandished some heavy-duty wire cutters. Without another word he cut Toffee free and shoved her backwards into our field, where she casually walked away as if nothing had happened.

'Thank you! I'm so sorry about that! I'll ask my friend to fix the fence! I'm so so sorry!' I blabbered.

'Nyaa,' he muttered. From his pocket he pulled out a ball of orange baler twine and with a few deft moves he fixed the fence. Then he stomped back off to his tractor and carried on with his day.

'What the hell to do about Toffee?' It was so stressful. Florence thought it was hilarious and she laughed her head off. 'I'm glad you find it funny. Oh heck look at the time. We've got to go now!'

I had to drop Florence at my parents' house and dash home to get ready for work. I was very relieved that it was Lady Alexa and not a non-horsey client. As soon as she walked in the door, she could tell I had a disaster to talk about.

'Spill the beans!' she chortled. 'I can tell from your expression that something truly ghastly has happened and I'll wager you've had nobody to talk to about it!'

'As usual, you're right.' I grimaced. 'But you aren't here to listen to my woes.'

'Nonsense! I insist. I've got plenty of time to listen to you before my massage.' She made herself comfy on the couch and I could tell she genuinely did want to know so out it all came. Sapna's nasty behaviour and Toffee's dreadful antics.

'Oh good gracious!' gasped Alexa. 'She sounds like a piece of work! Was she like that right from the start?'

'No she seemed like a really nice person at first but we only saw her for riding and moving those annoying ponies. Maybe this is the real her?' I wondered.

'And how awkward that your rent has been doubled. You're in a cleft stick as they say.' Lady Alexa was very sympathetic. 'I wonder how old she is?'

'How old? That's an odd thing to wonder about!'

'Not really.' Alexa looked thoughtful. 'How old does she look?'

'Around fifty-ish,' I replied, wondering what relevance her age could possibly have.

'Ah I may be correct then,' declared Alexa, folding her arms and smiling triumphantly.

'Correct about what?' I had no idea what she was talking about.

'Menopause!'

'Menopause?'

'Yes! Surely you know what it is?' laughed Alexa.

'Well yes, but what has that got to do with how bloody awful she is?'

'I think it could be her hormones. Menopause can turn even the kindest woman in the world into a raving monster.' Alexa nodded. 'There was a woman at a yard I was at who was the sweetest person you could hope to meet. Then menopause struck and whoomf, she was venomous!'

'Hmm. I wonder if you're right?' I hadn't thought much about menopause as it wasn't in my near future, but I had heard that it could cause awful moods. 'I'll see what Jack thinks.'

'As for Toffee.' Alexa grinned. 'What a monkey! She needs to go to a professional trainer if you two can't cope with her. She's only going to get worse.'

'Yes,' I sighed. 'Jack has been trying to sell her but nobody has replied to the adverts. She won't want to spend money on a trainer though.'

'Well nobody will want to buy a problem pony. Would you?' Alexa shrugged. I had to admit there was no way in the world I'd want to buy Toffee. I sighed and commenced the massage. It wasn't easy to focus on my work with thoughts of Sapna and Toffee buzzing around my brain like a couple of annoying bluebottles.

Chapter 23

'Hurry up, Mummy! We're going to be late!' Florence shouted. I was busy washing fox poo off Wrexford's neck and shoulder where he had joyfully rolled in it. He stank beyond description and nothing I used seem to be getting it off. There was nothing I could do except dry him off and shut him in his crate in the kitchen. I left a note telling James to finish cleaning him up.

'Poo! Wrexford!' Florence laughed. 'You are a stinky boy!'

'He most certainly is, so he can't come with today unfortunately,' I replied, sternly. I was sick of washing fox poo off Wrexford. He always seemed to do it when I had other important things to do. Florence had her riding lesson to get to so we dashed out of the house and set off for Think Like a Pony.

The riding school was set in the midst of glorious countryside and the drive through the pretty lanes was very soothing. I loved seeing all the beautiful, rolling fields filled with cows and sheep. It was quite a horsey area too so there was always a handful of riders along the way. We arrived in good time for Florence to help groom and tack up and even that was a lesson in itself for me. There was no battle to get the bridle on, the pony almost did it himself. With Poppy I had to stretch right up to get the reins over her head but it seemed that Florence had been taught how to get the pony to lower his head for her. I was very impressed.

'Good morning!' greeted Lynn, the owner of the riding school. 'You've got me today, Florence, so I want to see some good riding.' Lynn winked and led the way into the outdoor arena where two other girls were having lessons.

'Right, Florence, let's get cracking! What's the first thing you should do before mounting your pony?' Lynn stood with her hands on her hips and a broad smile on her face.

'We need to make sure he's comfortable and that we are connected,' said Florence with great confidence.

'Very good,' Lynn nodded. 'Let's check his tack is on properly first.' Lynn had a thorough look. 'Excellent! Now let's see you walk him around to see how connected you are.' Florence walked and halted, changed direction and did a bit of trotting with the pony.

'Oh very good.' Lynn grinned. 'Right, on you get!'

Florence mounted and set off walking under Lynn's eagle eye.

'Watch out for that pony, Florence, you're going to crash! Turn him away!' yelled Lynn as Florence almost barged into one of the other girls but managed to avoid collision at the last moment.

'Florence what are you doing, girl?' Lynn laughed. 'Get that pony under control!' For some reason, the pony kept going back over to the other pony and Florence seemed to be at a loss as to how to stop him.

'You've got to really believe in yourself, Florence!' shouted Lynn. 'I believe in you! Do you believe in you?' Florence didn't look too sure. Lynn walked over and led Florence and her pony away from the other lesson. 'Right let's do an exercise. Off you get!' Florence dismounted.

'When you were walking it was all going well wasn't it? So let's do that again.' Florence began walking with the pony. 'He's going where you decide, very good! Let's see a trot!' Florence and the pony trotted around and all the time he was listening to her and not attempting to go to the other pony.

'So Florence, what were you doing differently when you were riding?' asked Lynn.

'Er, I don't know.' Florence thought very hard.

'I think you were all up in the air! Get back on and imagine that you are walking on the ground next to him, leading him.' Florence mounted again and began walking.

'Very good! Imagine you are leading him where you want him to go!' Florence smiled as she realised she had gained control of the pony. 'You are the leader even when you are sitting on his back. It's very easy to give up leadership when you sit down on a pony but remember – just because you're sitting down it doesn't mean you're resting!'

I loved watching Florence's lessons. I learned so much about my own sorry state of riding and knew I needed to practise more of what I had learned in Wales. It was so similar – the use of energy and intention.

I wish I could bring Toffee here to get trained.

God what a brilliant idea! Maybe I should ask?

She'll say no I bet.

But it's worth asking isn't it? Just do it!

'Ok, Florence! Off you get now. You can untack him and give him lots of cuddles for being such a good boy.' The half hour had flown by and Lynn walked over to me.

'She's a grand little rider.' She smiled. 'She's really coming on.'

'Yes I'm very proud of her. I love all the psychology that you weave into the lessons. It's such a brilliant way of teaching.'

'It's much needed too,' agreed Lynn. 'The old-fashioned methods should be consigned to history as far as I'm concerned.' I couldn't agree more as I remembered my own childhood lessons, in which we were often shouted at to 'Give it a kick and tell it to get on!' by various ignorant and jaded instructors. I shuddered at the memories. The ponies had been treated like machines. We were never encouraged to give them cuddles and massages like they did at Think Like a Pony or even care if the saddle fit properly.

'Do you ever take ponies in for training?' I blurted, dreading the inevitable no.

'Yes we do. Would you like some help with Toffee?' asked Lynn. I almost fell over with shock as I was not expecting that.

'How do you know about Toffee?'

'Florence has told us all about her,' laughed Lynn. I had no idea she'd mentioned it. 'Is she your pony now? Florence said you were going to buy her from your friend?'

'Did she?' I grimaced. 'No, she's still my friend's pony but I have a feeling that I will have to buy her eventually.'

'Florence will go nuts if you don't,' chuckled Lynn. 'And worst-case scenario is she can live and work here.'

'Wow! Really?' I was stunned at the concept.

'Yes, we need a few more ponies now that we're expanding the centre, so if Toffee does well with her training, she can stay here. It's probably a better place for Flo to ride too because she'll have instructors around and other kids too.'

'I'm absolutely lost for words!' I burst into tears.

'Oh dear!' Lynn said and gave me a hug. 'What's all this about?'

'It's been so stressful dealing with Toffee! We have no idea about how to train a youngster. And even though she's a really big pain in the bum, I don't want her to be sold to a total stranger and end up in an awful home.' I suddenly realised how responsible I felt for Toffee's life even though she didn't belong to me.

'Well you can stop worrying now.' Lynn smiled. 'We'll help sort her out and she can stay here.' Florence overheard the conversation and whooped with joy.

'I'd better tell James!' I realised. 'Yikes!'

'He probably knew this was going to happen.' Lynn winked and had to go and greet her next pupil.

'I'll tell Jack first,' I said to Florence, who was madly dancing a jig of excitement. I pulled my phone out of my pocket and with shaky hands sent Jack a text.

'Oh my God brilliant! Chat later, I'm working!' she replied immediately.

'Heck! How are we going to tell Daddy?' I asked Florence.

'We'll just tell him,' she replied matter-of-factly.

'Hmm yes,' I agreed, doubtfully.

The drive home was not as relaxing as the drive there had been. *What have I done? James will go mad! Too late now though!* My mind went round and round interminably. It was excruciating. But it was too late. I couldn't go back on it or Florence would be devastated. However, the thought of being responsible for another horse made me want to vomit.

James was sitting at the kitchen table drinking a glass of water when we arrived home and I wanted to plan how I was going to break the news about Toffee.

'Guess what, Daddy? Mummy bought Toffee! Yay!' Florence couldn't contain her excitement as she danced round and round the kitchen. Water spurted out of James's mouth and his eyes almost popped out of his head.

'You did what?' he shouted.

'Er yes, I seem to have bought Toffee.' I winced.

'Why?' he demanded in horror.

'I don't know! It just sort of happened all by itself,' I squeaked.

How did it happen? I furiously tried to work out how I had got from wondering if they'd train her to saying I would buy her.

'Well you're going to have to un-buy her!' yelled James, his face bright red. 'We cannot afford two horses!'

'I hate you!' Florence burst into tears and ran out of the room.

I collapsed on a chair and hung my head in my hands. 'What have I done?'

James sat down next to me and said nothing. The silence was sharp. 'I don't know what to do about it!' I wailed.

James breathed deeply. 'How much would it cost to keep Toffee? She needs training and she needs a saddle and food and God knows what else.'

'Well it won't really cost anything except the tack because Lynn said they'll train her and she can live and work there so Florence can ride her in a safer place.'

'Oh! Why didn't you tell me that at first? If she can live there that's fine!'

'Really? You're alright with buying her and the tack?' I couldn't believe my ears.

'Well I'm not one hundred percent alright with it but it won't be much will it?' asked James.

'No, not for a small pony. A few hundred pounds?' I had no idea but I assumed it would be less than Poppy's saddle and bridle had been.

'Ok well that won't break the bank. And she can definitely live at Think Like a Pony?'

'Yes because they're expanding and need more ponies.'

'Well that's great. We'd better tell Florence.' James stood up and called Florence.

'Go away! I hate you!' she shouted. We went upstairs and found her with her head buried in Wrexford's sleeping body. He was oblivious to the whole situation and was happily dreaming and farting. The stench was almost chewable.

'You can have Toffee,' sighed James as he knelt down next to Florence.

'Really?' Florence turned her head round cautiously.

'Yes, but she has to live at Think Like a Pony and you can ride her there,' he replied.

'Yay! I'm going to tell all my friends!' Florence jumped up and gave us both a hug before dashing out of the house to tell her friend who lived across the road.

'Thank God for that.' I sat down, quickly regretted the decision and leaped to my feet. 'Why does this dog's bum always smell? And he still stinks of fox poo! He's going in the bath.'

It was actually quite relaxing to wash Wrexford after all that stress. He loved lying in the warm water while I massaged baby shampoo into his fur.

'I never wanted one horse and now we've got two,' laughed James, sitting on the edge of the bath. 'One of my patients warned me that this would happen and I said absolutely not a chance. She's going to laugh her head off when I tell her.'

'Well at least that's Florence's birthday present sorted.' I grimaced.

'Ha yes and her Christmas present.' James nodded.

'I'm so relieved. I was so worried about what might happen to Toffee,' I sighed. 'Florence is having the childhood I wish I'd had.'

'Yes, she's very lucky isn't she?' agreed James. 'When I was little I used to pretend I was a knight, cantering around on a horse.'

'What?' I spluttered. 'You never told me that!'

'Yes,' James laughed, immersed in his memories. 'My mum even made me a costume!'

'Wow!' I couldn't believe my ears. 'Did you ever have riding lessons then?'

'No but I rode my friend's pony that lived in a field at the bottom of our road.'

'How come you've never told me this?' I was amazed.

'Don't know. It's not something I've thought about until now.'

'Do you want to ride Poppy?' I asked. 'Or Buddy?'

'Yeah ok, I'll have a go.'

You could have knocked me down with a feather. 'No way! Right we're going to do that now!'

I hastily rinsed and dried Wrexford, who looked very disgruntled to have had his bath cut short. Then we collected Florence from her friend's house and drove to the field.

'Is Daddy really going to ride?' asked Florence, wide-eyed.

'Yes!' I had to see it to believe it.

Poppy was enjoying a little snooze when we arrived and looked rather peeved to have been so rudely interrupted. Her face spoke a thousand words when she realised who was going to be riding her. She looked for all the world as if she said, 'You can't be serious?'

'Do you know how to mount?' I asked, suddenly feeling a bit nervous.

'Of course I do,' scoffed James, thrusting his foot in the stirrup and springing effortlessly from the ground into the saddle as if he'd ridden every day of his life. I was shocked. Then I realised I was a bit annoyed.

How the hell did he do that at his age? I can't do that and I ride all the time!

'Mounting blocks are for sissies,' laughed James as he asked Poppy to walk on all the way around the top half of the field. His seat was perfect. He was a natural. I couldn't get my head round what I was seeing.

'That's enough for me,' said James as he leaped off.

'I'm lost for words! I can't believe you never told me you can ride horses.' I was stunned beyond description.

'Well done, Daddy!' Florence clapped her hands. 'Would you like a horse too?'

'Absolutely not,' he replied emphatically. 'I don't really feel interested in riding any more.'

'Well I just don't know what to say!' I was speechless. It really surprised me to think he'd had this secret for so long. It was very peculiar.

'I see that none of you noticed Toffee was out on the road because one of you idiots had left the gate wide open,' came a scathing voice. We turned in unison to see Sapna in the carpark leading Toffee in by her forelock. 'She was in the hedge on the corner.'

'Oh my God!' I hadn't noticed the gates were both open or Toffee sneaking out. In fact it dawned on me that Toffee hadn't been in the way while we were tacking up Poppy like she usually was. 'Thank God you found her!'

'Yes, thank God. But what are you going to do with her?' demanded Sapna. 'It can't go on. She's too much for you and Jack.

Neither of you know what you're doing. It's ridiculous for people like you to have a young pony!'

'You don't need to worry about it any more,' interjected James. 'She's going to Florence's riding school.'

'Finally, someone with sense! I'll be glad to see the back of her.' And with that she marched straight past us into the field shelter.

'What's her problem?' asked James raising his eyebrows.

'She's not very nice,' I said.

'She's rude!' said James looking over at the shelter. 'You need to sort that out.'

'Hmm,' I agreed. We swiftly untacked Poppy and got back in the car to go. None of us bothered to call out 'goodbye' to Sapna.

Why does she make me feel so afraid? I wondered, staring out of the window blankly as the scenery flashed past.

What am I so worried about? Why don't I tell her to stop being so nasty? I'm an adult now. Why do I feel so nervous? I need to speak to Jack about her.

My mind whirred round and round for the entire journey home and continued into the evening. It got distracted eventually by the mundanities of life and then I remembered James's amazing riding ability that he'd kept hidden. It was bizarre to have learned something new about him after having spent so many years together.

Chapter 24

It was the day for Poppy to have her follow-up with Marcus and I was anxious to get everything out of the way because I was dying to see him again and learn more about his extraordinary gift. I had to get Florence to school which was always an irritating experience due to the onslaught of cars all searching for parking spaces. What annoyed me the most was that most of these people lived close enough for their children to walk to school. We lived much further away so I had no choice but to drive. I always ended up muttering various oaths under my breath as I joined in the battle for the place to park.

Once I had escaped the maelstrom, I had to walk the dog. This time I kept my eagle eye on him and as soon as he showed any signs of even thinking about rolling in fox poo, I was on him like a ton of bricks. Poor Wrexford. He loved to make himself as foul-smelling as possible but I had had enough of cleaning him up. Miraculously, we finally managed to do a walk which didn't end in the need for a bath. So a quick dash to the shops then home to feed the dog and shove some laundry in the machine and then fly like the wind up to the field.

As soon as I turned onto our lane, my stomach began churning in exactly the same way as it had done all those years ago when I was terrified of going to school.

This is ridiculous! Get a grip!

I don't know why I'm so nervous. What's the worst she can do?

I felt sick and my hands became horribly clammy. I was annoyed with myself because usually I loved to turn off the main

road and look at all the beautiful fields. It was my time to relax
and let go of tension but instead I was full of dread. I breathed a
huge sigh of relief when I pulled into the layby and saw that the
carpark was locked so nobody was there.

The first, and only, horse to greet me was Velvet. She was
waiting by the gate as if she had known I was on my way and she
made a little rumbly sound.

'Hello, Velvet!' I smiled as I got out of my car and skipped
over to give her a kiss. 'It's so lovely to see you!' Velvet looked
sublimely happy as I gave her a stroke and told her how beautiful
she was. She really was a stunning horse and her dark coat was
wonderfully glossy in the morning sunlight.

'I've got to get Poppy ready for her session with Marcus,' I
said to Velvet. 'Oh God! Where's Toffee now?' I scanned the field
but couldn't see her. It dawned on me that Toffee was now my
responsibility. It was a heavy and unpleasant feeling.

Why did I say I'd buy her? What happens if Lynn changes her mind?

Other people would be ok about having two horses. Why am I
filled with dread? What the heck is wrong with me?

A nudge on my shoulder made me jump out of my skin. It was
Toffee appearing from God only knows where.

'Oh thank goodness,' I breathed a sigh of relief and marched
over to get Poppy. Toffee came with, which irritated Poppy and
made it very difficult to get her headcollar on.

'Toffee go away!' I implored to no avail. She just looked at me
blankly. I pushed on her chest to try to get her to go back. It was
like trying to move a mountain. 'Toffee! Just move out of the way!'

In the end I managed to usher Poppy away and into the field
shelter where I was then able to put on her headcollar. I bent down

to pick up a brush and came face to nose with Toffee who had followed us and was peering inside the grooming kit. 'Seriously Toffee! Just go outside and play with something else!' I was exasperated. Toffee just didn't seem to understand that she was getting in the way and I had no idea how to move her. Grooming was almost impossible thanks to her standing so close to Poppy that it became too dangerous as Poppy was clearly extremely annoyed. In the end I had to admit total defeat and led Poppy out towards the carpark. Fortunately, something over in the hedge caught Toffee's attention and she trotted away.

'Thank God for that,' I muttered and finally managed to relax just as Marcus drove in.

'Hello!' he greeted with a cheery smile as he heaved himself out of his car. 'How are you?'

'Cross,' I laughed. 'Toffee is so annoying! I can't get her out of my way when I'm trying to do things with Poppy.'

'Oh dear,' chuckled Marcus. 'She's probably bored and needs another youngster to play with.'

'Yes,' I sighed. 'She definitely does!'

'So how is Poppy?' asked Marcus, giving her a stroke. 'She's looking well.'

'She's back to normal now,' I replied.

'Great! Let's see what comes up in the session.'

'You know all the stuff you told me, about her previous home?' I could no longer contain myself.

'Oh yes.' Marcus nodded.

'You were right! I found out loads about her first home and everything you said was true! How did you know?'

'Poppy told me.' He smiled.

'How?' I demanded. 'How can you hear a horse talking? Is it actual words?'

'Sometimes it's words but most of the time it's visual or a feeling of different types of energy,' replied Marcus as he set to work on Poppy's body.

'How do you mean by "energy and visual"?' I was very keen to know more.

'Well it's hard to describe really.'

'Try!' I insisted.

'Er, well I often feel an energy spike usually in my heart centre or third eye and it can feel good, bad or indifferent. Then it's as if a photograph has been put into my mind. Or it's a bit like a cinefilm sometimes, lots of moving images but with no sound.' Marcus smiled. 'At the moment, Poppy is showing me images of boxes.'

'Boxes?' I repeated.

'Yes. She's giving you very neatly wrapped, brown paper boxes as a gift. I'm asking her what's in the boxes but she won't say. It's private and only for you to know.'

'Wow! That's all so weird!'

'Yes,' he chuckled. 'She loves you and she really appreciates how much you care about her.' I felt quite choked up and under other circumstances I would have cried, but I didn't feel comfortable letting it all out in front of Marcus.

'I love her too. Very much,' I managed to say with a cough.

After a few minutes of silence, my emotions calmed and I felt more able to chat.

'I'd love to be able to hear her speaking,' I sighed. 'How do you do it? Can anyone learn how?'

'Yes.' Marcus nodded. 'You just have to be open minded and not expect it to happen immediately. The trick is to have a quiet brain. If you observe all your horses interacting in the field, you'll notice they don't make a sound – it's all based on intention, which begins as a feeling. If you tend to think a lot then it's not going to be easy for them to communicate with you because they use more feeling energy than thought energy.'

'I do think a lot.'

'Ok well, begin by standing with Poppy and relax your body and mind and just have the intention of being an open vessel ready to receive her messages. It might be an image in your mind or a feeling. You may even hear words. Just trust what you pick up but don't expect it to happen on the first attempt.'

'Ok.' I grinned. 'I'll give it a go!' I was excited to try it but also quite doubtful that I would be able to pick anything up.

'She's saying don't doubt yourself.' Marcus winked.

'No way!' I gasped. 'I was just thinking that I doubt I'll be able to do it!'

'I know! Poppy told me,' Marcus laughed.

'Oh my God that's incredible! How did she know what I was thinking?' I was stunned.

'Because you share a bubble,' he replied, matter-of-factly.

'What?' I had no idea what the heck he was talking about.

'You must have heard of auras?'

'Yes, but I don't one hundred percent know what they are,' I answered.

'It's an energy field,' explained Marcus. 'Every electrical item gives off an energy field and our brains and hearts are electrical organs so we have an electromagnetic energy around us.'

'Ok.' I nodded.

'I sometimes see it as a coloured light like a bubble,' he continued. 'When you are near Poppy your bubbles become one shared, yellow bubble around you both so she is able to sense everything about you including your thoughts and feelings.'

'Wow!' I was lost for words. I found it hard to digest such invisible concepts. 'It sounds completely mental.'

'It sounds absolutely bonkers doesn't it? But remember that the man who first predicted the existence of radio waves was assumed to be mad until it was proved real. Just because we can't understand things with our logical brain, doesn't mean it isn't fact.'

'Hmm. That's true,' I conceded. I stood quietly for the remainder of the session, trying to feel the connection between me and Poppy.

'Well, that's Poppy all done,' said John as he stood back and stretched his long arms up above his head. 'Let her have a couple of days to adjust before you try a short ride.'

'Ok.' I nodded. 'Thank you. It's been fascinating to hear all your weird spookiness.' I grinned.

'You're welcome! If you have any questions just give me a call.' Marcus smiled.

My one big question is what the heck to do with Toffee? I thought to myself as I led Poppy back into the field and noticed that Toffee was standing in one of the water troughs.

What is she doing now? For God's sake.

'Toffee! Get out of there!' I shouted. Toffee ignored me and continued splashing away, making all the water filthy and undrinkable. Buddy looked at me with imploring eyes as if to say, 'Please just take her away.'

'I know how you feel, Buddy,' I said as I patted him. 'Hopefully it won't be long before she can go to boarding school.'

The gate clanged and I looked round, dreading who it might be, but thank goodness it was Jack.

'Is the coast clear?' she yelled over to me.

'Yes!' I shouted.

'Thank God for that.' Jack grinned and leaped over the fence into the field. 'What the hell is Toffee doing now? Get out you idiot!' She gave her bum a poke with a stick and Toffee clambered out of the trough and trotted away. 'God she's a pain in the arse isn't she? When is she going to the riding school?'

'The sooner the better,' I replied. 'I'm waiting for the yard manager to text me with a date.'

'I'm so glad she's going to a good home though, even though she winds us all up.'

'Yes me too. They'll turn her into a great little pony I'm sure,' I agreed.

'Do you think they'll let us go and watch her training?' asked Jack. 'I'd love to learn what they do.'

'Me too! I'll ask Lynn.'

'Oh hell! Here comes trouble.' Jack nodded in the direction of the carpark where Sapna was opening the gate. She drove in and got out of her car then walked straight into the field shelter as if we weren't there and called Velvet over to her. Jack and I watched as she put Velvet's headcollar on and began to groom her.

'That's just so weird,' hissed Jack. 'What is wrong with her?'

'Lady Alexa wondered if it might be menopause hormones. What do you think? How old is she?' I whispered.

'She's older than me so yes it could be.'

'I remember one of my aunties went really weird years and years ago and my mum mentioned menopause, but I was too young to care about it at the time,' I said, suddenly remembering the drama of Aunty Pauline. 'She was so vicious. But then a few years later she was nice again and nobody mentioned it ever again.'

'I've not thought much about menopause but I suppose it's worth finding out about it as that's our next big adventure.' Jack smirked. 'I'll Google it later. I'm sure it'll make for some really fun reading.'

'She's like a thunder cloud, isn't she?' I mused.

'Yes. She really makes it a bad atmosphere here. I was going to go for a ride but all my gear's in the back of the shelter and I don't want to go anywhere near her. I'm gonna go home and come back later.' Jack almost tiptoed away and I wasn't far behind her.

This is utterly ridiculous! I fumed as I drove back home.

How can I allow this weird woman to make me feel so bad?

But it's not just me. Jack also feels bad and she's a tough woman!

I arrived home and made myself a cup of tea. I had no work booked in so there was plenty of time to read up about the menopause. I hadn't given it any thought whatsoever but Jack was right. That was our next big adventure and it always paid to be prepared.

Do I really want to know about this right now? I asked myself.

Yes! You need to be ready just in case.

God. Ok I'll look.

With a combination of dread and fascination, I sat down with my laptop and searched for information about the menopause. I remembered my mum vaguely complaining of hot sweats and headaches but she was a very stoic woman and that's about all she had said about it. She was the type of woman who just soldiered on.

What the heck? This sounds hellish!

Hot flushes! Vaginal dryness! Mood changes! Sleep problems! I shut my laptop.

I don't want to know!

Curiosity got the better of me though and I couldn't resist reading more. It was extremely depressing to read the almost endless list of ghastly symptoms. How can hormones, or the lack of, create such horrors? But it made me wonder if perhaps that was the reason why Sapna was such a horrible person to be around. There was no time left for reading more as school pickup dawned and I had to get going. My mind chewed over everything I'd read all the way to the school gates, but I soon forgot about it as I had to take Florence to the dentist.

Later that evening I was cooking dinner when my phone pinged.

'Hi Grace. We can come and collect Toffee next Thursday morning if that suits you?' It was the yard manager from the riding school.

The relief was immense. It was like a lead weight had been lifted from my shoulders and for the first time in a long time, I did some disco dancing in the kitchen.

Chapter 25

The more I read about the menopause and how awful it could be, the more I wondered why my mother had never really mentioned it that much. Or maybe that was the reason why she had chosen not to? I decided I would see if she would talk about it over a cup of tea. She was dropping something off for Florence so I invited her in and put the kettle on.

'Mum?' I began.

'Yes, love?'

'What was your menopause like?' I went straight to the point.

'Oh heck! What a question! I thought you were going to ask if I could babysit,' she laughed.

'No, I need to know about the menopause,' I replied, anxious to keep on topic.

'Gosh, I can't really remember it was so long ago.'

'Try and remember!'

'Well, it was hard to sleep, I know that much. I kept getting hot sweats through the night so I was always very tired and my brain felt like it was full of fog. That's when I started getting migraines too. And I vaguely remember that everything smelled too strong, you know, perfumes and such. Why do you need to know about menopause? You're not old enough for that surely?'

'Oh it's just this awful woman who owns Velvet. She's always angry and to be honest I dread going up to the field in case she's there. She's completely ruined my enjoyment of having a horse,' I explained.

'That's terrible! Would you like me to go and speak to her for you?'

'No Mum, it's ok, I can handle it.' My mum seemed to think I was still only six years old. 'Jack and I were just wondering if she's like that because of her hormones. She used to be a nice woman when we first met her.'

'Well, it could be if she's over fifty? Do you remember what happened to your Aunty Pauline? You might have been too young. Anyway, she had such a terrible time with her hormones. Can you remember?'

'Vaguely. I remember hearing Grandma saying not to talk about it.'

'Oh yes! Grandma was so embarrassed about it,' laughed my mum.

'Why? What was she like?' I was fascinated.

'Goodness! She was like a monster! And nobody could believe that sweet Pauline could be so nasty. I remember her pouring a large glass of red wine over Uncle Stanley's shirt in a restaurant in front of all the family!' My mum roared with laughter at the memory. 'Nobody said a word! They just carried on eating as if nothing had happened!' Tears rolled down her cheeks. 'It was so funny!'

'I sort of remember.' Little snippets of Aunty Pauline began popping up in the dark recesses of my mind.

'But then after a few years she calmed down and nobody's mentioned it since.' Mum sipped her tea. 'I'd better get going or your dad will wonder where I am.'

I watched my mum drive away and pondered further on the possibility of menopause being the cause of Sapna's atrocious behaviour.

She's either a psychopath and kept it hidden from us or her hormones are affecting her mind.

Or maybe she's just a total bitch?

Hmm yes she could just be an absolute cow and we are allowing her to ruin our lives.

Why are we tiptoeing around her? What is it about her that is making us unable to speak up? Bugger this. I'm going for a ride!

With a deep breath, I changed into my riding clothes and set off towards the field. I felt powerful and ready to tell Sapna to sort her attitude out.

I'm not tolerating this any longer! This is our field and she can go and find somewhere else to take her horse!

Oh God there's her car in the layby. My heart began to speed up and a sensation of nausea washed over me.

What should I do? I pulled in behind her car.

Just go in and do what you need to do and don't let her stop you!

Just at that moment, the gate opened and shut as Sapna came out clearly leaving.

Phew! Thank God for that. I wound my window down.

'Hi Sapna,' I called out with fake cheeriness. 'Would you mind leaving the gate open so I can drive in?'

'Do it yourself you lazy cow!' she snarled. I was stunned. Too stunned to know how to respond so I waited for her to get in her car and leave before I opened the gate and drove in.

'What an absolute bitch!' I said out loud to myself. 'That was completely unnecessary!' I felt shaky, which made me annoyed for allowing someone to make me feel so bad. I got out of my car and stood next to the fence for a while.

She is the most horrible person I've ever met! I can't cope with her any more. She has got to go!

But then we will have to pay all that rent.

Bugger that! Sapna is bloody awful! Why should we put up with her?

Just at that moment, Velvet came over to me and nuzzled my face.

'Your owner is vile,' I said to her as I stroked her soft nose. 'I feel sorry for you!' Velvet was such a lovely horse, I felt sad at the thought of her going anywhere else. 'If only Sapna didn't come up so often, then it would be fine.'

'Hellooo! Grace! Are you there?' came a yell from down the lane. I nearly jumped out of my skin.

'Er yes,' I replied, walking to the gate to have a look around.

'Denwyn won't move!' It was Wendy. 'It's taken ages to get him all the way here but now he won't budge at all and I don't want to get off again!'

'I'll lead him,' I laughed and jogged down the lane to where they were. 'You did well to get to here.'

'Well to be honest, I've been on and off like a yoyo. It's so annoying,' replied Wendy with great exasperation.

'Shall I get a lead rope and lead you back to the farm?' I volunteered.

'I'd love that but God, that's a bit embarrassing, isn't it?'

'It might be what he needs for a while until he gets used to going out alone though? And I could do with a walk after what's just happened,' I replied.

'What's just happened?' asked Wendy.

'I'll get a lead rope and tell you on the way.' I dashed back to the field shelter, grabbed a lead rope and hurried back to Denwyn and Wendy.

'Right, Denwyn! You're not on your own now so let's get walking!' Miraculously, Denwyn walked on nicely without me having to put any pressure on the rope at all.

'I think he just needs to build confidence slowly,' I said. 'It must help him to relax if there's someone by his head.'

'It's embarrassing though. But yes I think you're right.'

'I don't think it is. It's just training, look at it that way.'

'Yes that's true,' Wendy conceded. 'So, what's just happened with you?'

'Where to begin? You know we have Sapna paying us to look after her horse?'

'I've not met her but yes.' Wendy nodded.

'Well, she's an absolutely horrendously awful woman!'

'Oh no! Why?' Wendy asked wide-eyed.

'She's permanently angry and extremely rude and aggressive. I've never met anyone like her! Yet she seemed so nice at first.'

'That's weird. But I wonder, how old is she?' asked Wendy.

'Early fifties,' I replied.

'Could be the menopause do you think?' suggested Wendy.

'Well that's what someone else said and I have been reading up about it and she does fit in to the description but I don't know. Maybe it is?'

'If you've seen her being nice and now she's like that it could well be hormonal,' ventured Wendy. 'My sister-in-law had a total personality change when she started her menopause but she's on HRT now thank goodness and she's back to normal more or less.'

'Really? Maybe it is that then? But even so, I don't see why we should put up with that.'

'You need to talk to her about it. But you can only really talk to her when she's calm or she won't see reason,' Wendy advised.

'Since she arrived, I've never seen her not in a bad mood,' I sighed.

'That's a tough one. You won't be able to talk to her when she's angry. It'll make her worse.'

'She's so bad already I dread to think of her getting any worse,' I shuddered at the thought of it. We walked down the lane and eventually arrived at the farm.

'I'd love to be able to ride Denwyn down that bridle path alone. He won't even walk in-hand down there.'

'He might if I lead him?' I offered. 'I've got time to do a longer walk if you want to try it?'

'That would be great if you could.' Wendy grinned, urging Denwyn on. He didn't take much persuading with me at his head. He obviously wanted to go out and do things, he just needed the confidence of having a couple of people as support.

The bridle path was such a beautiful track, flanked by wild hedgerows of different species. Some holly, some hawthorn and lots of rambling roses. The heady scent of a random honeysuckle lifted my spirits and calmed my mind. Fields full of sheep added a pleasant soundtrack of 'baa' amidst the merry tweeting of birds and the occasional moo drifting through the air. There was nowhere else I would have wanted to be.

'God it's so lovely here, isn't it?' It was the first time I'd been on foot down the bridle path so I was able to see all the low growing tangle of vegetation which had lots of butterflies flitting around.

'Yes, we're so lucky to have this place to ride,' agreed Wendy. 'I really love those pine woods coming up round the corner. The smell reminds me of being on holiday in Cyprus.' We rounded the corner and the soft scent of pine filled the air. It was very 'holiday-ish'.

'Whoa!' yelled Wendy as Denwyn suddenly reared. His hooves

whistled over my head as they skimmed past me. I jumped backwards into a huge clump of nettles.

'Ow! Bloody hell!' I scrambled to my feet. 'What's spooking him?' Denwyn bucked and tried to spin round but Wendy held on and managed to calm him down.

'Denwyn! Settle down!' she commanded. 'What the heck was that about?' We scanned the area and saw nothing but Denwyn was still very unsettled and although he continued to walk his head was high and he kept neighing.

'Should we turn back?' I wondered.

'Maybe? I don't want him to get into bad habits of turning round when he wants to though,' replied Wendy nervously. 'I'm not happy though.'

'Do you want to get off but keep going this way?' I suggested.

'Not sure!'

'What the hell was that?' I jumped. Denwyn jumped and snorted.

'Oh my God! It's a pig!' gasped Wendy.

'It's three pigs! No it's five! Or is it six? Is that another one over there?' I couldn't believe my eyes. 'It's ok, Denwyn! It's just some pigs in the woods. What the heck are pigs doing in there?' I laughed and relaxed and that had a calming effect on Denwyn, who suddenly became interested instead of nervous.

'There's another two over there look! So I think that's seven?' Wendy was open mouthed, as was I.

'What should we do?' I wondered. 'We can't really leave them can we?'

'I don't know! Maybe they're happy in there? But no you're right we have to do something but what?'

'Er I have no idea whatsoever,' I replied completely perplexed. 'Here piggy piggy! Do you need to be rescued?' Bizarrely, they responded and came closer snorting and snuffling.

'Wow,' laughed Wendy. 'They're very tame! Aren't they little? They must be very young, or maybe it's a mini breed?' By now the pigs were pushing through the undergrowth to get closer to us.

'It's so weird!' The pigs seemed to have a leader who came right up to us to sniff us. Denwyn lowered his nose and joined in with the sniffing. 'He's good isn't he? If that was Poppy she'd be off like a shot into the next county.'

'Yes he's great with farm animals, thank goodness,' agreed Wendy. 'But I have no idea what we should do and I can't call Adam because he's at the cattle market today.'

'I suppose we could call the police?' I asked.

'Yeah good idea. Oh hang on! Is that? No surely it can't be?'

'What?' I didn't know what she was talking about until I followed her gaze. 'Wow! Yes it is!'

'Hello!' shouted Wendy, almost deafening me. She waved her arms at two police officers who were approaching further down the bridle path. 'Over here!'

'There are some pigs in the woods!' I shouted. The police began jogging towards us.

'Bloody hell,' panted one of them as they reached us, almost collapsing. 'We've been searching for those pigs! We thought it was a joke caller but then we got more messages about them so we thought we'd better investigate.'

'How many are there?' gasped the other one, also red in the face and out of breath.

'We've counted seven so far,' I replied. Doing a quick head count. 'Yes seven. No eight, oh blimey look there's another one!' There was indeed another pig nearby eating a bush.

'Well I'll be buggered,' said the first policeman shaking his head. 'What the hell are we meant to do about this?'

'That's what we were wondering. I have no idea.' I shrugged my shoulders.

'It's a serious offence to dump pigs if that's what has happened,' grumbled the second one. 'They're small, aren't they?'

'Yes we were just commenting on that.' Wendy nodded.

'In yesteryear there used to be special places for stray farm animals and owners would have to pay to get them back,' I remarked. 'I think they were called pinfolds.'

'We could do with one of those right now,' replied the first policeman. 'I'm going to have to call this in and see what we should do.' He unclipped his radio and began talking. 'We've found some stray pigs in woodland. What should we do about them?'

'Did you say pigs?' laughed the surprised voice on the other end.

'Yes pigs! Loads of small ones.'

'I've got absolutely no idea,' replied the voice. 'I'll have to ask someone. I'll get back to you.'

'Great,' said the exasperated policeman. 'Nobody knows what to do about these pigs!'

'I could ask Rob?' I suggested. 'He might know about it. He seems to know everything else that goes on around here.'

'Good. You call Rob, whoever he is.' The policeman nodded. 'Who is Rob?'

'He's a gamekeeper,' I replied as I looked for his number on my phone. Fortunately, he answered immediately. 'Hi, it's Grace! Do you know anything about some pigs in the woods on the bridle path behind Adam's farm?'

'Oh for God's sake is that where they are?' he spluttered.

'Whose pigs are they?' I asked.

'They belong to the estate. Some idiot left a gate open and they got out. There should be nine of them.'

'Oh dear,' I replied.

'What is it?'

'There's only eight here.'

'Bollocks. I'm on my way now. Don't let them go anywhere else!' Rob hung up.

'There's definitely only eight, isn't there?' I asked, scanning the woods.

'Yeah, just eight.' Wendy and both policemen nodded.

'Oh for God's sake!' erupted the second policeman, who clearly did not like pigs. 'Where are they going?'

We all watched in horror as the pigs decided it would be a great idea to explore the barley field next to the woods.

'Whose field is this?' I wondered, as the pigs began to tuck in with gusto.

'I think it's the estate's,' laughed Wendy, who was finding the whole scenario hilarious.

'Oh well it's their lookout then,' harumphed the policeman. All we could do was watch and pray that the pigs remained in the field and didn't decide to go further away.

'By the time Rob gets here there won't be much left of that crop,' declared the first policeman with his hands on his hips, shaking his head. We all nodded in agreement as we watched the almost total desecration of the field.

'They must be hungry,' I chuckled. 'Oh thank God, there he is!' Rob's quad bike appeared on the path at the opposite end of the field and he sped towards us.

'Oh bloody hell!' he shouted. 'How am I going to get them out of there?'

'Er, well they seem to be very hungry, so maybe offer them something tastier than barley?' I suggested.

'I've got some crisps!' offered Wendy, leaning over and rummaging around in her saddle bag. 'I brought them to entice Denwyn along. They're cheese and onion so they might like that flavour?'

'It's worth a try,' sighed Rob. 'I've got a trailer at the bottom of that field ready for them. We just need to get them there.'

'Well this is one to tell everyone back at the station, that's for sure. Come on then everybody, how are we going to do this?' The second policeman seemed to have cheered up a bit and appeared almost enthusiastic.

'I'll see if they like the smell of the crisps and if they do, I'll start walking and then if you can all create a barrier around them all and herd them onwards?' suggested Rob. He opened the crisps bag and strode into the field. It was very fortunate that the pigs were so friendly and they were soon snuffling around him, eager to gobble all the food.

'They like it.' He looked round and grinned. 'I'll try walking now.' Rob turned and walked away with the pigs all following him, shrieking and snorting.

'Brilliant,' laughed Wendy. 'I don't think he needs our help but I suppose we should make sure they get in the trailer.'

We all followed at a distance, trampling on the sad remains of the barley field and quite quickly reached the trailer. Rob chucked the bag of crisps inside and they all galloped in, almost crushing each other in their excitement to get the food.

'Well that was easy,' I breathed a sigh of relief as I had visions of this madness going on all day.

'I wonder where the other pig is, though?' said Wendy.

'Over there!' yelled the first policeman, who had spotted the errant pig in the hedgerow, watching us with suspicion.

'What's it doing?' I wondered. 'Why isn't it following its friends?'

'It's probably the wise one of the bunch,' Wendy chortled. 'Right, let's go and get it! Who's got a snack?' Unfortunately, nobody had any food on them and all the crisps were long gone.

'That pig looks like it knows we are wanting to get it,' I said. 'How are we going to entice it over here?'

'Oh hell,' said Rob. 'I've got no idea.'

'If you three stay here, we'll go over there and drive it towards you,' suggested the first policeman. 'Then you can catch it!'

'Yeah that should do it.' Rob nodded. The policemen set off towards the pig, making friendly noises so as not to scare it. But it wasn't an idiot. It knew exactly what was going on and it wasn't giving up its freedom lightly. In a flash, the pig turned tail and charged straight through the hedge and hurtled across the neighbouring field, at an unexpected pace for a barrel shaped animal with short legs. We watched it disappear through the hedge at the far end of that field.

'Wow!' I was impressed. 'Who knew pigs could run so fast?'

It suddenly dawned on Rob what was behind that hedge. 'It's heading for the set of Birkdale Farm!'

'Oh no! We'd better get over there then,' I replied, resigned to the fact I was involved with this charade until the bitter end.

'We'll leave you to it,' said the first policeman. 'We've got crime to fight!' and with that the pair of them hurried away.

'Get on!' Rob commanded, gesturing to his quad bike. 'Wendy, can you follow us? Might need Denwyn to help!'

'I'll try,' Wendy replied doubtfully. 'Come on, Denwyn, we're on a mission!'

Rob's quad bike stank of diesel and didn't go as fast as I was expecting but that wasn't such a bad thing as it meant that Denwyn was able to keep up. We finally rolled up to the entrance of the Birkdale Farm fake village film set and stopped.

'Have you got a pass?' enquired the security guard on the gate.

'No!' replied Rob. 'But we need to go in immediately!'

'I'm sorry, sir, but I can't let you in without a pass.'

'One of my pigs has got through the hedge onto the set so you really need to let me in!' insisted Rob.

'Well that's a new one,' laughed the security guard, shaking his head. 'Look, sir, as you can imagine we get a lot of fans trying to get in with all sorts of excuses and I'm afraid I'm not falling for your pig story!' The security guard picked up his radio and pressed a button.

'You alright there, Dipak?' came a voice over the radio. Dipak winked at us.

'Got some fans here trying to get in. They said one of their pigs has got through the hedge onto the set!' Dipak roared with laughter.

'Oh bloody hell! Send 'em through quick!' In the background, over the radio, we could hear shrieks.

'No way? I thought you were taking the piss!' exclaimed Dipak as he dashed into his hut to release the switch that would open the barrier.

'If only.' I grimaced. The barrier lifted, painfully slowly, and in we went.

'Now is not the time to graze!' yelled Wendy. I looked back to see that Denwyn had taken a fancy to some weeds by the edge of the road and was heartily snaffling them up. Wendy yanked on his reins and almost ended up falling off with the exertion. 'Denwyn! Come on!' Denwyn snorted his annoyance but finally complied.

'Bloody hell,' sighed Rob. 'Come on, Denwyn!'

The closer we got to the set, the louder the shouting became.

'Who the hell let a pig in here?' yelled an irate man's voice. 'Is this a joke?'

'Can someone get the pig out of the pub, this isn't funny!' shrieked a lady's voice.

'I hate pigs! Has it gone?' yelled someone else.

'No! It's in the pub!' someone replied.

'Oh my God!' I laughed. 'It's in the pub!'

'Yeah, I heard,' Rob said, clearly not very amused.

'Are you the owner of the pig?' shouted a security guard rushing over to us.

'Unfortunately, yes,' replied Rob.

'It's in the pub! Follow me!' The security guard hurried us down one of the realistic yet fake village lanes to the pub. 'It's gone in there and it's hiding behind the bar apparently.'

'You!' roared an aggressive voice. A short, stocky man wearing a cream, linen suit and a lilac neck scarf marched towards us. His face was bright red beneath his Panama hat. 'Are you the prankster who's let a pig into our set? I've got a good mind to report this to the police! I do not and I repeat *do not* like pigs or any other animal for that matter! Madam, can you kindly reverse your horse it's standing too close to me.' He shot an angry stare at Wendy, who really wasn't anywhere near him.

'Isn't this soap opera about farms?' I enquired, innocently.

'What's that got to do with it?' shouted the man rendering me speechless. 'Remove the pig immediately. You are interfering with my schedule!'

'I'm going to need to shut him in the pub and bring my trailer up here,' said Rob calmly, 'and I will need a very big piece of cheese or some other strong-smelling food.'

'Pardon?' the short man almost exploded. His eyes popped out very comically. 'You're asking us to delay our filming AND you want some food? Marian call the police I've had enough of this nonsense.' A youngish-looking, wispy blonde girl hurried over.

'Oh I don't think we need to call the police?' She spoke very softly with her head cocked sharply to one side. 'I'm sure it's all an accident, isn't it?'

'Yes!' spluttered Rob. 'We haven't done this on purpose, you bloody idiot. We've got other things to do as well. Close the pub doors and let me get my trailer and get me some food so I can lure him out!' I got off the quad and Rob drove away before anyone could respond.

'I'll be in my office!' bellowed the short, angry man. 'Call me when this pantomime is over!' He flounced off very dramatically. Marian breathed a sigh of relief and smiled weakly.

'Who's he?' I asked.

'He's one of the directors,' replied Marian apologetically.

'They're not all like that. He's just a little temperamental at times.'

'A little?' laughed Wendy.

'Hmm yes well you know how these types can be.' She blushed. 'Oh Zara, could you please get a big chunk of cheddar from the catering van?' Marian asked another wispy sort of a girl who was floating around nearby holding a clipboard. The girl trotted off and returned just at the same moment as Rob who had come back with his trailer full of pigs.

'Someone will need to keep these pigs in the trailer while I lure the one in the pub. Grace can you do that?' asked Rob.

'Er well I can try! Don't you think it would be safer to leave it closed until you get the other pig?'

'No. I need the ramp down now or we'll not get him in.'

'Denwyn might be good at that job?' suggested Wendy.

'Great stuff.' Rob shot her a thumbs-up, opened the trailer door, grabbed the cheese and walked purposefully over to the pub.

'Stay back!' I commanded as I parked myself on the trailer ramp and opened my arms wide. The pigs snorted loudly. It was very disconcerting. 'Wendy, bring Denwyn!' I squeaked.

Denwyn pawed the trailer ramp and lowered his head, snorting back at the pigs. He was very good. I was amazed at how confident he was with them. I knew that Poppy would absolutely never in a million years be able to do that. Suddenly a loud squeal alerted us all to the fact that the pig in the pub was on his way over.

'Thank bloody God they love food,' muttered Rob as he lured the pig to the trailer and led him up the ramp. We all breathed a sigh of relief and apologised to everyone nearby.

'Thanks for helping.' Rob grinned. 'I'd better get this lot back to where they belong.'

'Crikey! Look at the time!' I suddenly realised it was nearly school pickup. 'Come on, Denwyn!' We jogged all the way back to the farm and then I flew like the wind to our field, puffing and panting. By some miracle of fate I wasn't too late to collect Florence. She was playing with some friends in the playground thankfully.

What a day! I laughed to myself as I drove home.

Chapter 26

Thursday morning couldn't have come soon enough. The relief of Toffee being taken away for training was indescribable.

What happens if she behaves so badly that they send her back? My mind suddenly went into overdrive and my heart began beating ten to the dozen.

What if she just can't be trained?

I can't cope with a pony like Toffee! I'm not experienced enough!

'I'm here! Are you on your way?' My phone pinged, jolting me out of my worries. It was Jack. She was anxious to send Toffee off well so she had arrived early to give her a bath and hair brush.

'Coming now!' I hastily replied as I leaped into my car.

Bloody hell! I forgot to feed the dog! I scrambled back into the house.

Where the hell is the can opener? Who's moved it? Oh my God I haven't got time for ... oh it's there for God's sake. Who left it there? Stress anger bubbled up.

'Right! I'll see you later,' I said to Wrexford and ran out of the door.

What the hell? Traffic had built up down the main road and nothing was moving.

What's going on? Why is nothing moving? I craned my neck to see what was happening ahead but could see no reason for the hold up.

Oh my God! Move! Why are you all out on the road at this time of the day? Why aren't you all at work? I was furious.

Just get out of my way!

After what felt like an eternity, the traffic began moving again but my blood pressure was sky high. I tried some deep breathing, which slightly helped to take the edge off it, but it began to rocket the closer I got to the field.

I hope Sapna doesn't turn up. That's the last thing we need today.

Fortunately, there was no sign of her as I parked up in the layby and dashed over to the gate.

'God!' I panted. 'Everything is too stressful today!'

'Calm down, woman,' laughed Jack. 'Look how beautiful Toffee looks now that she's had a bath. Still can't get the grass stain off her knee but it's better than it was.' Toffee looked very pretty and ready for her new life, despite one pale green knee.

'You've done a great job.' I nodded approvingly. 'I can hear an engine! That might be them!' My heart leaped as I dashed over to check what was coming.

'Oh my God, it's Sapna!' I looked over at Jack with horror.

'Oh for God's sake.' Jack's face fell. 'That's all we bloody need. She can't park in here we need the space for the horse box.'

'Oh hell yes! I'll tell her.' I grimaced.

'Good luck!'

Sapna wound her window down and shouted, 'Can you mind out so I can drive in?'

'I'm really sorry but we need to keep the carpark clear for the horse box,' I replied with a pathetically apologetic voice.

Why did I apologise? I'm not sorry and she can piss off!

'Oh right. Fine.' Sapna reversed and parked behind our cars. Without even a hello, she stalked past us like a dark thunder cloud, into the field shelter and called Velvet over. For the first time ever, Velvet didn't respond. Instead, she walked past the field shelter and headed straight for me, making the lovely rumbly chuckling sound that she had begun to greet me with.

'Ah, hello, Velvet.' I gave her a stroke. Sapna glared at me. 'I think your mummy wants to see you.' The atmosphere was leaden.

'Velvet!' called Sapna, sharply. But Velvet chose to completely ignore her and instead rubbed her face on my chest. Jack stifled a nervous laugh. Without a word, Sapna strode over to Velvet, put her headcollar on and marched her back to the shelter.

'Oh my God!' mouthed Jack, raising her eyebrows. Luckily, the horsebox arrived just at that moment so all thoughts of Sapna disappeared.

'Good morning!' greeted Lynn, who was driving. Another lady was in the passenger seat as a back-up in case they had trouble loading Toffee. Suddenly I felt a surge of emotion and I realised I couldn't speak or I would cry.

Oh my good God! What the hell is wrong with me? I swallowed hard.

Fortunately, Jack took over and helped load Toffee, which involved quite a lot of commotion so I didn't have to say anything.

'Right!' said Jack when the ramp was closed. We could hear Toffee banging about and neighing. She was obviously very disturbed by the situation. 'We'll follow behind you and then Toffee will see us at the other end and hopefully will settle easier.'

'Good idea,' agreed Lynn, giving a thumbs-up.

Poppy sauntered over to watch the proceedings and looked for all the world as if she was saying, 'Goodbye and good riddance! Don't come back!' She actually had a little smile on her face and she breathed deeply, flaring her giant nostrils.

'I can see you're very happy about this,' I said to Poppy as we watched the horse box reverse slowly out of the carpark. I like to imagine that she replied with, 'I most certainly am!' Buddy nodded his approval too and was probably saying similar comments to Poppy, but I didn't have time to hang around. Jack and I hurried to her van and followed the horse box down the winding country lanes to Think Like a Pony.

'I feel a bit emotional,' admitted Jack, wiping a tear from her eye.

'Me too.' I nodded. 'It's odd because Toffee is so annoying and stressful. Why am I feeling sad?'

'We must have got used to having her around even though she's a pain in the arse,' laughed Jack. 'I'm looking forward to seeing the place after hearing so much about it from Flo. It's gorgeous round here, isn't it? Can you imagine being able to afford a house like that?' I looked out at the enormous country manor we were passing and agreed it would be amazing.

'But you'd have to have staff though,' I remarked. 'Or you'd spend all day, every day, cleaning the damn thing and can you imagine keeping up to that garden? What a nightmare! And God forbid you forget where you left your car keys. It would take at least a week to find them. No thanks, I don't want to live there.'

'I don't want to live there now either, you nutter!' laughed Jack. 'Wow! Is this the place?' The horsebox had pulled in to Think Like a Pony.

'Yes. It's beautiful, isn't it?' I sighed, wishing that we could have a top of the range equestrian facility. 'Now this is where I'd like to live.'

'Oh yes, this would be perfect. Is that the arena over there? It's massive, isn't it? Wow! God I would love to have a place like this.'

We stepped out of the van into the warm sunshine. The sky was blue with the occasional cotton-wool cloud floating leisurely along and the delicious smell of stables wafted through the air. It took me right back to my childhood where the only place I was truly happy was at the riding school.

'Ok, everyone, stand back,' announced Lynn. 'Let's release the tiger!' She unhooked the pins that kept the ramp shut and carefully lowered it to the ground. Poor Toffee looked very discombobulated and rather sweaty from the stress of the experience. Lynn untied her lead rope and led her out of the horsebox. As soon as Toffee saw us, she neighed and dashed straight for us.

'Hello Toffee!' I gave her a cuddle. She blew in my face, clearly relieved to see me.

'Don't worry, Toffee, you've come to a five-star luxury resort.' Jack grinned giving her a pat. 'Wish I could live here!'

'It's great, isn't it?' Lynn nodded, smiling. 'This is my dream come true.'

'I bet,' laughed Jack. 'Can we have a look around?'

'Yes of course! Let's get Toffee settled first and I'll give you a guided tour.' Lynn led us to a large field full of ponies and inside was a temporary pen where Toffee could safely get to know her new herd.

'Come on, Toffee! This is your new home now,' I implored as she planted all of her feet and refused to move. 'I think she knows she's come to school and can't get away with murder any more!'

'Come on, Toffee,' encouraged Jack, scratching her shoulder. 'I promise you'll love it here!' Toffee still refused to budge.

'There's only one thing for it,' said Lynn, firmly taking hold of the lead rope. I was ready to watch some horsemanship in action and was interested to see how Lynn would manage a situation like this because I had no idea what to do. Jack and I stood back to watch the master in action.

'Come on, Toffee, stop messing around.' Lynn rummaged around in her pocket and pulled out a packet of mints. Toffee walked on instantly and happily went into her new pen. 'If in doubt, get the mints out! It's one of my favourite mottoes,' she laughed.

'Oh,' I laughed. 'I was expecting you to do some horse whispery type stuff!'

'Sometimes it's easier to use bribery, like with toddlers.' She winked. 'But seriously, I think you should both come and be involved with Toffee's training. It will be good for you to see what we do here.'

'What do you do here?' asked Jack with interest.

'We do all sorts.' Lynn grinned. 'I'll show you around.' Lynn led us to an indoor school where there were large, educational posters on the wall about ponies and how they think and respond.

'This is where we usually start with youngsters who have never been near a pony before. We teach them all about how to handle them safely and respectfully. Then when the child is aware of all of that, we go out into the big arena.' Lynn led us outside, through a courtyard and over to the enviable outdoor arena.

'This is where we begin the ridden work but it's more than just riding, as Grace has already seen from Florence's lessons. We teach the kids how to feel the energy of their ponies and how our energy and emotion impacts on the behaviour of the pony.'

'Wow,' said Jack. 'I'd love to know all that stuff.'

'Well you'll learn it here with Toffee. We also work with

kids with special needs and kids from unpleasant backgrounds. Our work helps them to control their own antisocial behaviour and become more confident. They're then able to make good relationships with other people and go on to become valuable members of society.'

'That sounds brilliant,' said Jack.

'It really is.' I nodded. 'I can't wait to learn it myself instead of just watching Florence.'

'Well let's let Toffee settle in for a couple of weeks first and then we'll begin. Is that ok with you both?' asked Lynn, looking through her diary to put a date in for the first session.

'Great,' we both agreed.

We drove back to the field in silence. Both of us digesting the events of the morning.

'Oh God,' murmured Jack, as we rounded the bend just before our field. 'Sapna's still here. What is she doing? I wanted to go for a ride.'

'Oh no,' I sighed. 'I thought she'd have gone by now.'

Jack parked in the layby and we both almost tiptoed to the gate. Without a word, Sapna walked past us, got in her car and left.

'Thank the Lord for that!' announced Jack. She fanned herself and sat down on the mounting block. 'It's hot isn't it?'

'It is,' I agreed and went to get my water bottle. 'What are we going to do about Sapna?'

'Ignore her?' suggested Jack.

'I suppose in a way we are ignoring her, but it's so uncomfortable, isn't it? I dread her being here and it's ruining the joy of having our own place.'

'Yeah, I know. I dread coming here now. It's shit, isn't it?' agreed Jack.

'What shall we do?'

'I don't know. She's so weird! Have you ever met anyone like her since not being at school? She is literally the classroom bitch, isn't she?'

'Yes, she really is and I don't know why I can't stand up to her. Why do I freeze?'

'It's awful, isn't it? I'm the same. She needs to go to Think Like a Pony and learn how to stop her antisocial behaviour.' Jack laughed her head off.

'You're not wrong,' I agreed. 'I'd better go. Got to work now. You enjoy your ride.'

I drove home, pondering on the concept of Sapna attending Think Like a Pony. If only we could get her to go. I was sure it would help her to see what a total cow she was and learn how to be nicer. But the reality was, neither Jack nor I would ever dare to suggest such a thing for fear of having our heads bitten off.

Chapter 27

Two weeks seemed to fly by in a whirlwind of ordinary life stuff and suddenly it was time to attend the training of Toffee – a much-needed experience for all concerned. The sun was shining in the deep blue, cloudless sky and the emerald grass of the pastureland seemed to almost glow. It was a perfect day to be outside.

'She's not in her pen any more,' I noticed as we walked over to the pony field. 'Toffee!' I called out and she trotted over to see us.

'She jumped out of her pen the first night,' laughed Lynn who had walked over to greet us. 'We put her back in and she jumped straight out again so we let her stay in with her new mates.'

'Sounds about right for Toffee,' muttered Jack, giving her a pat. 'You've got to behave yourself or you'll get expelled.'

Lynn put Toffee's headcollar on and led us all in to the large, outdoor arena.

'The first thing we do when training a horse is to establish clear boundaries,' explained Lynn. 'This isn't to be dominant or bossy, it's to help create a clear and safe relationship.'

Jack and I nodded dumbly.

'I have to be honest,' I piped up. 'I don't really know what you meant just then.'

'I'm glad you said that, Grace.' Lynn smiled. 'Because it's no good me jabbering away if you don't understand what I'm saying. So please always ask.'

'Yeah,' Jack chimed in. 'I didn't understand it either.'

'Ok ladies, I'll make it clearer. This young pony, like a human child, is testing the boundaries of every horse and every person she meets. She wants to know where she stands and what she can get away with. Imagine you've got a sandwich and you're just about to eat it and then I come along and grab it. How would you feel?'

'Shocked! And then really pissed off!'

Jack nodded in agreement. 'I'd think you were a bit mad.'

'Right,' said Lynn. 'And if you didn't stop me, I'd do it again and again and then I'd do worse things! In not much time, the relationship would be very unpleasant and out of balance.'

'It would be awful.' I nodded.

'Exactly. Well imagine half a ton of horse completely disrespecting you. It would be more than awful, it would be very dangerous. Not only because the animal could injure you but imagine if you were out riding in the countryside. Something might scare the horse. This horse doesn't respect you so she isn't going to listen to you when you try to stop her from running away and injuring herself and other people.'

'Ah yes!'

'So step one is to teach the horse where the stop line is. Let's just have a look at the bigger ponies in the next field for a few moments.' Lynn invited us to follow her to the fence and we all stood and watched the big ponies grazing. 'Ok, so watch the brown one there. He's walking. Can you see from his body language he's very intent on going to that patch of long grass over in the corner. Now wait and see what the grey pony does who's already eating there.'

'Wow! How did he move her away without touching her?'

'And from so far away?' added Jack.

'Because he felt so strongly that that was what he intended to do,' explained Lynn. 'And the grey doesn't feel as strong within herself so she yielded. Let's go back to where we were and we will practise.' Lynn walked back into the middle of the arena and unclipped Toffee's lead rope. 'We'll do this without Toffee first. Ok Grace, I want you to think about yourself in a kind and loving way. Really focus on your positive attributes. Are you ready? Here I come!' Lynn marched right up to me and easily pushed me backwards.

'Yikes!' I squeaked.

'Now where is your mind, Gracie? It's not focussed! What were you thinking about?'

'I was trying to think of something positive about myself but I didn't know what.'

'I see. So that tells me that you doubt yourself quite deeply. I can see a lot of positive things about you. I know that you work hard at making your animals as comfortable as possible, which is a credit to you. How lovely that you cared so much about Toffee that you were willing to buy her so she could have a good life. Really be aware of how kind you are and how lucky any animal is to be yours.'

I pondered on her thoughts and nodded. I did care very deeply about the well-being of all animals. 'Ok I'm ready,' I grinned.

'Ooh that's better,' laughed Lynn as she pushed me. 'You didn't even budge. Well done! Do you see how powerful our thoughts are about ourselves?'

'I'm amazed!'

'So Jack, it's your turn now. Think about something really good about yourself.'

Lynn made Jack walk backwards easily and then she went through the process of visualisation with Jack until she could no longer take the ground on which she stood.

'It's a fun way of demonstrating how horses, and indeed all herbivores, interact. They use the silent yet super-powerful language of the mind. Now our human brains are so cluttered up with all the jobs we need to get done that we have lost the power that comes from a clear and focussed mind. Horses don't do that. They live in the moment. They are only thinking about now. What do I need to do now? They aren't thinking "I need to get the shopping done by five and collect so and so from Cubs so that I can then have the dinner in the oven before seven." They're thinking one thought at a time and it's only about what is happening in that present moment.'

Lynn gave us a few moments to digest that information before continuing.

'When the mind is focussed it harnesses the power of the heart to create a tangible sensation that can affect any person or animal nearby. This is how the brown pony moved the grey without a word and without touch. We, as humans, need to remember how to use our hearts and minds more effectively. So let's return to Toffee's training.' Lynn collected Toffee from where she was scratching herself on the fence and brought her into the centre of the arena.

'I need Toffee to know that I am a very kind person but I will not allow her to walk all over me. She needs to know that what I say is important because I value myself. She needs to respect my boundaries. So many people say "my horse needs to learn respect" but they don't seem to realise that respect has to be earned by being firm but kind. Kindness is vital in all aspects of animal training.' Lynn walked Toffee around in a circle and then asked her to walk backwards by shaking the lead rope. Toffee didn't budge. 'Now as you can see, she either doesn't understand what I'm asking her to do or she does understand but doesn't want to walk backwards.'

'She's too pig-headed to take instructions,' muttered Jack under her breath.

'So I need to make my intention clearer and use more belly button power,' continued Lynn. 'This is where you imagine you have a lightsabre jetting out from your belly button and when you really focus on that imagery it helps the horse to know where you want to direct them. So I am going to focus on my self-worth and generate a feeling of love in my heart for myself and Toffee. And then I am going to visualise where I want her to move – out of my space using my lightsabre.'

'I bet it won't make any difference,' whispered Jack.

'Wow!' I gasped as Toffee walked backwards. 'It worked!'

'Well I'll be buggered,' said Jack. 'Can't believe it!'

'It's good isn't it?' laughed Lynn. 'Ok now let's teach Toffee where my boundary is. My boundary is an arm's length all around me. That's my energy bubble and Toffee is not allowed inside my energy bubble unless I invite her in. And this is how it works within the horse herd too.'

My ears pricked up at this statement and my mind went back to my time in Wales where Julie had taught me about energy bubbles.

'I'm visualising my bubble as a solid glass ball all around me then I'm going to put a little bit of pressure on the lead rope to encourage Toffee to walk towards me. When she reaches my boundary, I will use a clear hand signal to stop her,' explained Lynn.

'Good luck with that,' muttered Jack.

'Walk on, Toffee!' instructed Lynn. 'And whoa!' Toffee stopped an arm's length away from Lynn. 'Now that was very good so I will reward her by stepping closer to her and I'll give her a scratch. It's vital to reward even a small try. This will encourage them to want to try harder next time.'

'That's great!' said Jack, raising her eyebrows.

'I'm amazed,' I laughed. 'I didn't think she'd stop.'

'It's all very simple and straightforward, really,' said Lynn. 'You just have to be very clear with your intentions and value yourself.' One of the other instructors entered the arena leading a small, sandy-coloured pony.

'Shall I just do some lunging with him?' she asked Lynn.

'That's good timing,' replied Lynn. 'I think I'll borrow him for this training session so the ladies have a pony each. Can you go and exercise one of the others instead? Thanks!' The instructor handed the pony over to Lynn and left the arena.

'Ok so Grace, you take Toffee, and Jack you can have this little man. He's called Biscuit. Biscuit is a fully trained pony but he's very sensitive and strong minded so he won't make it easy for you.' She winked. We both took hold of the lead ropes and Lynn spent a few moments ensuring we relaxed our shoulders and released any tension in our arms and hands.

'If you're tense you'll block the communication between you and the pony,' she explained. 'Right, are you both ready?' We nodded.

'We'll begin with you walking the ponies around the arena to create a connection first, so off you go,' Lynn instructed. 'Very good. Now come back into the centre, but don't stand too close to each other and whoa! Excellent. Ok, now turn to stand facing your pony's head and then ask them to go backwards.'

I turned to face Toffee and waggled the lead rope. She looked at me with a blank expression on her face. 'Come on, Toffee, go back,' I implored and waggled the rope again.

'You've got to really mean it, Gracie!' called Lynn. 'Use that belly button lightsabre!' I visualised a purple light blazing out of my belly button but still Toffee didn't budge. Glancing over to Jack I was relieved to notice she was having similar trouble with Biscuit. 'Increase the power behind your intention ladies! And wave an arm at them too!' Jack and I waved our arms and both ponies stepped back a little.

'Well that's a good start.' Lynn smiled. 'Now really ramp up that power of intention. Make them walk back a few more steps. Come on, really focus!' It took a lot of effort to get a few more steps out of both ponies. 'Very good! Now rest a moment.' Jack and I stood still, awaiting the next instruction.

'What I'd like you to do next is to put some gentle pressure on the lead rope, tell them to walk on and when they're an arm's length in front of you, stop your ponies by putting your hand up and saying "whoa". Are you ready? Ok!'

I pulled slightly on the rope and said, 'Walk on!' briskly. Toffee walked towards me. 'Whoa!' I commanded and put my hand up. Toffee bashed right into me. 'Ow, you little bugger!' Jack had a similar experience with Biscuit.

'Never mind,' laughed Lynn. 'Let's try again and this time really focus hard on where you want them to stop.'

I took a deep breath and sent Toffee backwards, which took several attempts, and then asked her to walk towards me. Once again, both Toffee and Biscuit walked right up to our bodies. We tried a few more times and each time was an abysmal failure.

'Let's take a short break and relax,' said Lynn, turning the ponies loose.

'Why can't we do this? You make it look so easy!'

'Yeah!' agreed Jack. 'How is it that you can do it and we can't? It looks like such a basic thing to do.'

'I think these ponies are showing up a bigger issue for the both of you,' replied Lynn.

'What do you mean?' I asked, perplexed.

'Well let's consider what it is we are attempting to do. The exercise was all about stopping the pony from stepping across a boundary. The boundary was wherever you decided it to be. From observing what kept happening, it appears that you don't have any boundaries. So the next step would be to look at your daily life and see where you allow people to take advantage of you.'

'Nobody takes advantage of me!' responded Jack haughtily.

'Me neither,' I agreed, thinking about how I no longer allowed my massage clients to mess me about.

'Really?' enquired Lynn. 'Let's try a little exercise. I'd like you both to take a deep breath and close your eyes.' Jack looked sceptical but gave it a go. I had no idea why we were being asked to do this but I closed my eyes and took a deep breath anyway.

'Now,' continued Lynn softly. 'Can you think of anyone who is unsettling you?'

'Sapna!' said Jack and I almost simultaneously, opening our eyes wide.

'Who's Sapna?' asked Lynn.

'She keeps her horse at our place and she's an absolute bitch,' replied Jack.

'She's horrendous,' I agreed and poured out the whole situation to Lynn. 'And for some weird reason we just don't seem able to say anything back to her,' I concluded and Jack nodded in agreement.

'Now that's very interesting,' said Lynn, narrowing her eyes as if deep in thought. 'There was something that you kept repeating throughout that story. It was the word school bully.'

'She flipping is a school bully,' blustered Jack.

'Right.' Lynn nodded. 'May I ask were either of you bullied at school?'

'Yes,' I admitted, red-faced. 'There was a really horrible girl in my class that made me feel scared of going to school every day. She didn't do anything physical like hit me or anything it was all just psychological stuff.'

'Same here,' mumbled Jack. 'There was a girl in my class who was a complete and utter bitch from hell.'

'I see.' Lynn nodded. 'Can I ask, did either of you tell your parents about it at the time?'

'I did eventually, but it was only after it reached a big crisis point,' I replied, biting my lip.

'That's terribly sad, Grace,' said Lynn. 'It sounds like it must have been extremely stressful. How did your parents react?'

'Well I can remember my mum was very shocked and sad. I can't remember how my dad reacted. Then my mum became furious so she took me out of school immediately and I went to another school. But then there was another horrible girl at that school too who made me feel afraid so moving didn't make it better.' Painful memories began to surface and my eyes filled with tears. Lynn put a comforting hand on my shoulder.

'What a horrible time it must have been. May I ask, what was your mum like in general?' asked Lynn, handing me a tissue from her pocket. I wiped my eyes and sniffed.

'She was very loving throughout my childhood,' I replied. 'She still is. But a bit overprotective really and she still treats me as if I'm too young to be able to do things for myself.'

'Right, that's interesting,' said Lynn and she gave me a hug. Then she turned to Jack. 'How about you, Jack? What happened with your school bully?'

Jack screwed her face up, remembering her time at school. 'The girl always used to take the piss out of my clothes and my hairstyles. She was really nasty and made everyone else laugh at me too. But I couldn't tell my parents. My dad worked away a lot and my mum was too busy looking after all of us. I've got seven brothers so there's no way she would have been able to listen.'

'That's very sad that you felt she was too busy. How long did it go on for?'

'Oh God, years! All through school. I dreaded going every day.' Jack coughed and wiped some tears from her eyes. 'What a bitch!'

'Yes,' agreed Lynn, quietly nodding. She handed Jack a tissue. 'It's no wonder that Sapna is triggering such a reaction in the both of you after those experiences. I'd like to try something that I feel will help you to cope with her. Would you like to give it a go?'

'Yes please,' I replied.

'I'll try anything,' agreed Jack. 'We can't go on like this, dreading to bump into her.'

'Great stuff.' Lynn smiled. 'Have either of you heard about the inner child theory?'

'No.' I shook my head.

'Well they say that within us all lives our eternal inner child. It's the younger version of ourselves that holds the traumas of childhood that need to be healed. It doesn't necessarily mean a massively serious experience, it can be any incident in our childhood that affected us. An incident in which we were not helped by the adults. Now this can translate in a few different ways. Sometimes we aren't helped because sadly some parents just don't care. Sometimes we aren't listened to by busy parents. Sometimes we aren't helped because we aren't ever shown that we can be brave and do things for ourselves. So Jack, you didn't feel that your mum had time to listen to you. And Grace, your mum took you away from the problem but didn't empower you by teaching you that you can be strong enough to defend yourself from the bully and so it repeated in the next school.'

Jack and I nodded quietly as we ruminated on what Lynn had just said.

'So what happens is,' continued Lynn, 'when we come across situations later in life that resemble the same childhood incidents, we react in a similar way that we did all those years ago. They say it's the inner child alerting us to something that needs to be healed.'

'It really does feel that way. In fact, I have to admit I've been feeling a bit childish ever since I bought Poppy and even more so since we took on the field.'

'Really?' asked Jack. 'Why?'

'I just don't feel capable of being able to cope with the responsibility of it all,' I replied, my cheeks flushed crimson red and emotions bubbled up again. 'I'm embarrassed about it!'

'Try not to feel ashamed about how you feel, Grace,' said Lynn kindly. 'I'm not surprised you feel that way if your mum protected you too much.'

'Well now that we know about this inner child thing, how do we sort it out?' wondered Jack, who always liked a practical remedy.

'We are going to do an exercise,' explained Lynn. 'First of all, I'd like you both to release tension by rolling your shoulders and shaking your arms.' We did as instructed, then continued releasing tension from our bodies by shaking our legs and turning our ankles from one side to another. It was quite odd but felt great afterwards.

'Excellent. Now stand comfortably and close your eyes and take a few deep breaths,' continued Lynn. 'I'm going to ask you to access your memories. Are you ready?' We both nodded.

'Ok great. Can you remember a specific incident involving the bully? The first thing that comes to mind is perfect,' said Lynn softly and calmly. We both nodded.

'Now really picture the scene as vividly as you can,' she continued. 'Remember everything that happened, all the emotions.'

Tears streamed down my cheeks as I immersed myself in memories that I had shut away for so many years.

'That's such a babyish watch,' laughed the girl. 'Who wears a Snoopy watch at our age? Grace, you're such a big baby!'

My throat felt like it had filled with gravel and my heart began beating faster. I loved my new watch. It had a red leather strap and a picture of Snoopy in the watch face and it had been a birthday present from my parents, which had cost them a lot of money.

'It's so cheap and tacky,' she continued. 'Look at Grace's baby watch, everyone! I think we should give it to someone in nursery, don't you?' All the other girls tittered and giggled. In a flash, the girl ripped the watch off my wrist and threw it to another girl, who threw it to someone else, and so it went on with me feebly trying to catch it until a teacher came in and stopped it.

I can't take this any more, I said to myself. The teacher allowed me to go to the toilet and nobody noticed as I walked out of school and took myself home.

The sadness had grown over the years and felt like a lead weight in my chest, the burden of which was now too heavy to carry. I heard no sounds, even though there were cars driving along the roads. I felt no sense of the wind on my face or even the air temperature. Everything had become like a dream, a nothingness. The physical world had come to a stop as I put one foot in front of the other and found myself walking into the house. Nobody was in. My mind was completely silent and my heart as still as a stone as I opened the bottle of painkillers and one after another swallowed them all, very matter-of-factly.

I walked upstairs to my room and lay down on the bed.

Oh shit! I'm going to die! Panic suddenly set in and I sat bolt upright. Everything felt cold and my heart began racing.

Tell a neighbour immediately, said a strangely deep voice that came through my mind. It was like a man's voice.

I ran out of the house and went across the road to the old lady who lived opposite. She was always very kind. She would know what to do.

My memory went blank and then I found myself lying on a hospital bed.

'Come on, love, you've got to swallow this tube,' said a kind but firm voice. The tube was ridged and it scraped my throat as they pushed it down into my stomach. I retched and tried to pull it out but someone grabbed my hand.

'It's in!'

'Ok love, this will feel weird but it's just water so don't worry!'

A sensation of cold hit my stomach and then it all came up and out.

'Well done, love, you're doing great.'

Chapter 28

'Now,' said Lynn quietly, jolting me back to the present moment. 'I'd like you to freeze frame that memory of you as a child with the bully and nod when you've done it.'

My memory rewound to the moment where the girl took my watch.

'And now visualise yourself as an adult walking into that scene and nod when you have done it.'

Suddenly I saw the current grown-up me walking into the classroom.

'Now, allow the child version of you to see the adult version of you and nod when you've done that.'

In my mind's eye the younger me caught sight of the older me and a strong feeling of surprise welled up in my chest.

'Ok, now allow your younger self to tell your adult self what you need from them,' instructed Lynn.

I need help! squealed little me from the depths of my soul.

I can help you to stop this girl from being such a bitch! replied the powerful, adult me. *I am right next to you and you can tell her anything you want to say without any fear.*

I can't! I'm too scared!

You can do it! I'm right here and I have absolute faith in you. You are strong!

Suddenly the memory changed. Little me grabbed the watch and punched the girl in the mouth and she fell backwards onto the floor.

I hate you! You are the nastiest girl in the world and if you ever come near me again, I will tear your ugly eyes out! little me shouted at the bully and then kicked her in her chest. In my mind's eye the bully curled into a ball and begged for mercy.

Never come anywhere near me again! And the same goes for all you other stupid cows, do you understand?

I saw all the other girls nod and look afraid.

Wow! Well done, little Grace! Adult me was very proud. *You can tell all bullies to sod off out of your life now!*

The vision melted away and I opened my eyes feeling invincible.

'Wow!' I gasped, shaking. 'I literally feel like I am a different person.'

'Me too.' Jack smiled, wiping the tears from her eyes.

'It's a very powerful thing.' Lynn nodded, handing us both tissues. 'I'll let you recover and then I'll explain the science behind it.'

Jack and I wiped our eyes and blew our snotty noses. Then we automatically began moving our legs as if to ground ourselves once more and Lynn passed us a couple of water bottles she had handy. Drinking seemed to help bring me fully back into the present moment.

'You're the only people I've done this with,' explained Lynn, 'because it's not something I do myself as a teacher here. But I went through this method of clearing historical issues with a friend who's learning how to be a therapist and I was amazed at how quickly it transformed my way of being.'

'I really enjoyed doing that,' I sighed, feeling as if a huge weight had been lifted from the depths of my soul.

'I'm so pleased.' Lynn smiled. 'The theory behind it is that we can be our own parents and say the things we had needed to hear as children. It makes a real change in how our brains function and respond to new events.'

'Right, I think I can feel that. I do feel as if what I imagined was what really happened.'

'Yes that's exactly it. They say that if you visualise something with deep emotions, it's as real to your brain as it would be in real life.'

I was amazed by such a concept.

'In my mind, I spoke to myself as if I was my own mum and then I punched the girl in the face,' said Jack. 'I'm really surprised at how I actually feel better just from imagining that.'

'It's very effective, isn't it?' agreed Lynn. 'So now if you're ready we will go through the next part of the process. We'll sit down for this bit, I think. You both look a bit wobbly.'

Jack and I nodded. We were very wobbly after such a powerful experience and it was a pleasant relief to go and sit down on a few portable mounting blocks in the corner of the arena.

'Bullies can only harm us if we somehow feel less than them,' explained Lynn. 'Remember how the brown pony made the grey pony move away from the grass she was eating? That right there is the clearest demonstration of how someone who believes themselves to be powerful can move someone who is in agreement with that. The grey pony agreed that the brown pony was more powerful than her so she moved.'

Lynn quietly let us consider that statement for a few moments before continuing.

'If you begin to make a conscious effort to think positive thoughts about yourselves, you'll both transform in a way you can't imagine now. Love is a powerful tool and yet we are never taught to love and value ourselves as much as we are expected to love and value others.'

'That's true.' I nodded, thinking back to my childhood in which I was taught to always put other people's needs before my own.

'You have as much value as anyone else and you deserve to be able to live your lives without being spoken to so rudely by someone who has come into your space. It's time to create an aura of power around yourselves that Sapna will feel, and this is how we do it. Wait here, I'll be as quick as a flash!' Lynn trotted off to her house and returned holding a small mirror.

'Now I want you to watch closely what I am about to do, ok? This is a wonderful positive affirmation by Louise Hay.' She looked at herself in the mirror and cleared her throat. 'I completely love and approve of myself exactly as I am and I speak up for myself with ease.'

Jack opened her mouth to say something but no words came out.

'I realise that looks a bit odd.' Lynn smiled. 'But the more you tell your brain that you love yourself and that you can speak up for yourself, the more it will believe it. The brain is no different to a computer. Whatever you tell it to do, it will do.'

'I can't imagine saying that to myself.' I squirmed at the mere thought of it.

'I found it uncomfortable at first too but in time the feeling changes and after a while it makes you feel powerful. Powerful in a good way. It won't make you egotistical if that's what you're worried about. It will bolster your self-esteem and help you to boundary bad behaviour. The more you feel self-worth the more you will emanate an intangible aura of strength that will command respect.'

'I do like the sound of that, but I'd feel a bit of a prat to say that in the mirror,' admitted Jack.

'Just try it. You've got nothing to lose and everything to gain,' insisted Lynn.

'Ok,' I mumbled as I took the mirror and cleared my throat.

'We'll say it together,' said Lynn. 'I completely love and approve of myself exactly as I am and I speak up for myself with ease.'

'God it feels so weird!' I squeaked.

'Yes it will at first but after a few days it won't. Let's say it again. Jack you join in too.'

Jack and I repeated the mantra with red faces and in very quiet voices.

'Louder, ladies! Say it like you mean it!'

We increased the volume and forced ourselves to say it again.

'And even louder this time!' Lynn grinned.

'I completely love and approve of myself exactly as I am and I speak up for myself with ease!' I declared loudly.

'Excellent! Keep it up. Let's say it a few more times!'

After ten more repetitions we were shouting it as loudly as we could, much to the bemusement of Toffee and Biscuit, who had wandered over to see what was wrong with us. But I had begun to enjoy it and I could feel that it was something my heart and mind desperately needed as much as a plant needs water. This simple mantra felt like something I should have been saying all of my life.

'Well done, both of you. What I suggest you do now is say it twenty times every morning and night, each day for two weeks, then come back and repeat this exercise with the ponies,' said Lynn. 'Remember it has to be done while looking in the mirror and you have to say it out loud so that your brain actually hears it. I like to call it the mirror mantra.'

'Ok.' We both nodded.

The session finished, we led the ponies back to their field and turned them loose. Jack and I then walked back to the carpark in a bit of a daze.

'Well I wasn't expecting that,' I said with a deep sigh.

'Me neither,' agreed Jack. 'I can't even describe how I'm feeling now. But the more I think about it, the more it really makes a lot of sense. I'm going to feel like a bit of a twit saying that sentence out loud into a mirror every day but I'm going to do it.'

'Yes, me too.'

Jack drove us back to the field and we both almost tumbled out of her van into the carpark.

'I feel completely wiped out,' I murmured, sitting down on the grass, idly stroking the clover and enjoying the warmth of the sun on my head.

Jack sat down next to me and yawned. 'I actually wanted to kill myself when I was at school, you know. But I didn't want to upset my mum so I didn't do it.'

'I did try to kill myself,' I admitted and looked up at the clouds.

'No way, really? That's terrible! You must have felt awful! What did you do?'

'I took an overdose of painkillers but as soon as I'd done it I regretted it. Ended up having my stomach pumped, which was absolutely horrific, and then I had to see a psychiatrist for a few years.'

'Wow! I'm shocked. I don't know what to say. Poor you, how bloody awful. And your poor mum, she's so sweet. How did she cope with that?'

'I still feel guilty about my mum when I remember what I did.'

'Don't feel guilty. You were in a mess, obviously. I bet your mum felt guilty though too.'

'Yes she did and I think that's what I found the hardest. It wasn't her fault that I chose to not tell her what was happening. And when I think back now as an adult, I really can't understand why I didn't tell anyone. Why did I bottle it all up and then try and kill myself?'

'I don't think you can ever understand what a child's mind does, so don't tie yourself up in knots about it. Young people just don't think sensibly. They blow things up out of all proportion it's as simple as that.'

'True. My mind was very different to how it is now. The psychiatrist was so rubbish! All he did was give me various anti-depressants and asked me how I felt, but there was never any practical guidance like what we just did with Lynn. That's the sort of thing I needed.'

'I suppose in our day it was all about tablets wasn't it?'

'Yes. I'm amazed I managed to get through my life to adulthood when I think back to how depressed I was. But things got better naturally until recently. Louise began to trigger it at the old yard.'

'God yes, she was a cow, wasn't she? She always made me feel like I was a piece of dirt on her perfect boot.' Jack screwed her face up as if recalling a painful memory.

'Really? You always seemed as if you didn't get bothered by her.'

'I'm just good at hiding how I feel.' Jack smirked. 'It's how I coped with my school bully. But I feel sad because apart from you and Jan from Valerie's yard, I don't feel comfortable being friendly with anyone just in case.'

'How do you mean? Just in case of what?'

'Well the bully from my school had been my best friend for years when we were little. It was when we were about twelve that she turned into the bitch from hell, so I do feel afraid about opening up to people now.'

'God! I'm not surprised. That's horrible. That happened to James too. His best friend at school became a bully to him. It must be more common than we hear about. I hope this mirror mantra helps you to feel better about accepting friendships in future.'

'Me too.' Jack nodded. 'I feel that it will. If I ever see your bully I'll give her a right crack! You could have died and I'd never have met you!' Jack's eyes filled with tears and for once she didn't try to hide them. I cried too at the thought of her once-best-friend treating her so badly.

'I'll give you a hug, but don't expect it to happen again,' laughed Jack. I laughed too as I received the first and last hug from Jack.

'Let's really make a big effort to do this mirror work,' I said. 'We both deserve to feel better and not be treated like shit ever again.'

'Yes you're right. It's time we put the past well and truly behind us.'

I drove home extra slowly because I was feeling so peculiar. It was as if I'd been carrying a sack full of sadness around with me all my life that I had become so used to that I had ceased noticing it and now finally I had been shown how to let it go. I was amazed that something that had happened during childhood could still shape my responses to the present situation with Sapna and all the new responsibilities I'd taken on. But I smiled to myself as I realised what a relief to know that Florence was learning all about self-awareness at Think Like a Pony and how she would never be the victim of bullying ever again.

Chapter 29

I awoke to the sound of my phone pinging. It was Jack. 'Have you practiced your mantra this morning? I've done mine!'

'I'm still in bed,' I replied, astonished at her unusual level of keenness.

'You lazy cow! Get on with it, woman! I'll see you later.'

I yawned and rolled out of bed. I had the luxury of not having to do the school run that morning because Florence had had a sleepover at Grandma and Grandad's house so there was only Wrexford to deal with.

'I completely love and approve of myself exactly as I am and I speak up for myself with ease,' I said out loud to myself in the bathroom mirror.

God, what a weird thing to say.

Just do it! You know it will help!

'I completely love and approve of myself exactly as I am and I speak up for myself with ease.'

This is extremely bizarre.

Shut up and get on with it! My inner parent had developed a similar tone to Lynn.

'I completely love and approve of myself exactly as I am and I speak up for myself with ease,' I repeated it twenty times. By the tenth repetition it was beginning to feel less ridiculous and by the time I'd reached the last one I felt more comfortable saying it. I texted Jack to let her know I'd completed the task and she replied with a thumbs-up emoji. My phone pinged again.

'Your bloody ginger horse has been in my garden all night,

neighing. I haven't had a wink of sleep! Come and sort it out now. It's driving me mad!' messaged the landlord.

'Oh for God's sake!' I huffed out loud and replied to his message. 'Why didn't you let her out last night?'

'I couldn't be bothered to get out of bed,' he replied.

'Well you can't complain about it then!' I text back.

Oh my God! What have I just done! I can't believe I said that to him he'll go mad and kick us off! I felt sick with worry and my heart began to pound.

'Ha! Yeah I suppose you're right!' came his response.

'Wow,' I said out loud to myself and then I let him know I was on my way over.

I can't believe I got away with saying that to him. It must be that mantra?

I hurriedly sorted the dog out and thanked the universe that he was a whippet. Wrexford was very happy to zoom around the garden after a ball for ten minutes and then go back to his luxury, fluffy bed for several hours. He whined at me a few times because I hadn't covered him correctly with his blanket and his pillow wasn't entirely at the right angle but eventually everything was to his satisfaction and I was able to get going.

Sure enough, when I arrived at the field, I could hear the unmistakable neigh of Poppy, who was still in their garden.

Why has he not bothered to let her out? I fumed as I marched across to the rickety old gate that separated his garden from the field.

Oh for God's sake! I chuntered as it almost came off in my hand.

'Why are you neighing?' I asked as I observed Poppy. She looked extremely happy, wandering around eating various delicious fruits from their mini garden orchard and then every now and again she'd let out a loud neigh. 'I think you're just letting everyone else know that you're in an all-inclusive resort enjoying the endless buffet! I might join you actually.' I couldn't resist picking a juicy, blush pear and biting into it.

'The pair of you are bloody thieves!' shouted the landlord, who had sneaked up behind me. 'She's decimated my crop! I've a good mind to sue you!'

'You won't get far with that, you daft bugger. Look at your ridiculous gate!' I gestured to the dilapidated gate that was forlornly hanging off its hinges.

Oh my God, what have I just said?

Roger took a sharp intake of breath and his cheeks flushed red. 'Ha! You're right I do need to fix that gate. He's a lovely horse, isn't he? What's his name?'

'She's called Poppy,' I breathed a sigh of relief.

'Well she can have as many apples and pears as she likes. We don't bother eating them anyway, Valentina prefers to get fruit from Waitrose,' he replied, patting Poppy's sleek neck.

'Why? These are delicious!' I waved the pear under his nose.

'Is it? I've never tried them.' He picked a pear and inspected it suspiciously as if it might poison him.

'Seriously? That's crazy.' I couldn't believe my ears. 'Try it!' Roger bit into the pear slowly and thoughtfully. He raised his eyebrows in surprise.

'You're right! That's lovely, isn't it?'

'Yes and it's free and doesn't come in a horrible plastic carton.'

'I'll tell Valentina to try them.' He nodded.

'You're an odd guy you know,' I blurted bravely before I could stop myself.

'Am I? In what way?' asked Roger congenially.

'Sometimes you're really angry and shouty and then sometimes you're really friendly. Why are you so changeable?'

Silence.

Oh shit! I've gone too far!

Roger breathed deeply and pulled a face.

Oh God! My heart sped up.

'Well,' he replied staring up at the sky and twiddling his thumbs, 'I suppose I was expecting you to be like the previous tenant who never paid so I was primed for a problem.' He nodded as if he was happy with that explanation.

'Well as you can see, we are not like her and in fact we have improved your land by treating your ragwort, so really you should be paying us.' I was suddenly feeling very daring.

'Ha! You can have some apples and pears.' He picked an apple and handed it to me. 'There you go, don't say I never give you anything.' We both laughed and things felt more comfortable between us.

'I'd better get her out of here before she explodes,' I said as Poppy helped herself to a few more pears.

'Yes, I'd better get back to work,' sighed Roger and he wandered back towards his house.

'Come on, greedy guts,' I said to Poppy as I put her headcollar on. 'You've eaten enough fruit for a lifetime. I hope you don't get ill.' It suddenly dawned on me that eating so much fruit might actually be a bad thing for a horse. I dragged her away from the orchard before she could snaffle any more.

'I wondered where you were,' greeted Jack as we walked through the gate back into the field.

'Poppy had been in their garden through the night and I think they'll all end up getting in if we don't do anything with that awful gate.' I explained.

'Another job,' sighed Jack. 'He should be paying us!'

'That's what I literally just said to him.'

'No way! You never did?' Jack's jaw dropped open.

'I did! I was feeling brave,' I chuckled.

'Must be that mirror mantra! It's gone to your head already.' Jack grinned. 'I'll go and get some baler twine and just tie it shut for now.' She walked over to her van while I checked the pulses in Poppy's 'ankles' to check if she had any sign of laminitis after all that sugary fruit. Fortunately, all was ok in that department.

'Don't do it again!' I chided and turned her loose.

'Hope this will be enough,' muttered Jack as she unravelled a messy clump of orange twine. 'Oh God here comes trouble.' I looked over and noticed the gate opening. It was Sapna. Jack raised her eyebrows at me and we both watched her drive in. As usual she got out of her car, ignored us and stomped into the field shelter with a face like thunder.

'Come on!' I said to Jack and began walking over to her.

'Grace!' she hissed. 'What are you doing?'

'I've had enough of this,' I replied and marched into the shelter.

I vaguely heard Jack whisper, 'Do you think it's wise? It's only day one of the mantra!' but something significant had altered deep within the core of my being.

'Sapna! We need to talk!' I boomed with a volume that surprised me.

'Oh!' she replied, startled.

'We can't tolerate your rude behaviour any more. It's extremely childish and if you've got a problem with us both then I think the adult thing to do is to talk about it. So, what is your problem?' For the first time in a long time, I felt extremely calm.

'I'm so sorry!' Sapna suddenly burst into tears.

'Oh shit!' exclaimed Jack, completely stunned, as was I. There was an awkward moment in which Jack and I exchanged shocked expressions because neither of us knew what to do. I realised it was down to me to step in.

'What's wrong?' I asked, in a quieter voice and rummaged in my pocket for a tissue. Luckily there was a clean one so I handed it to her.

'Thanks,' she mumbled and blew her nose nosily. 'I don't know what's wrong with me. I just feel so enraged all the time. Like even tiny things flip me out and I just shout at everyone! I've been told to have some time off work and I've only just been transferred to this practice because I was being such a cow in the previous one.' She shook her head and looked genuinely mortified. 'I could lose my job!'

'Oh nightmare,' replied Jack, grimacing.

'Have you been to a doctor?' I asked kindly. 'We were wondering if it might be hormonal? Could it be that do you think?'

'Yeah, I think you might be right.' Sapna nodded. 'I suppose I'm at that age where it could be menopause. I had been thinking about it but I suppose I didn't want to admit it. Women's things is just not something we talk about in my family. I think I do need to see a doctor before I get sacked. I'm so very sorry that I've been so nasty. And I'm really grateful that you've come to talk to me. I've been feeling so lonely.' Suddenly she burst into deep, convulsive sobs. Jack looked mortified and pulled a face which clearly said *what the hell?* I gave Sapna a hug and she seemed to be grateful for it because she relaxed and hugged me back.

'Shall we call your GP now and get you an appointment?' I asked when she'd calmed down. 'You might feel better knowing you've got that sorted out.'

'Yes that's a good idea,' she sniffed. We stood with her while she made the call and miraculously, she managed to not only get through to the surgery in less than five minutes but because she was crying they gave her an appointment for later at the end of the day.

'Wow!' said Jack. 'That's a miracle. How on earth did you manage that? I can never get an appointment with my doctor.'

'It's the magic of the universe,' I laughed.

'Ha, yes!' agreed Sapna. 'I feel so much better for talking. I'm so ashamed of how I've been. Can we start again? I'd love to get to know your horses a bit more too,' she said as Poppy came into the shelter.

'Poppy's been eating apples and pears in the landlord's garden all night so now I'm worried about her getting laminitis,' I suddenly remembered.

'Oh no! I'll check her over.' Sapna went into work mode and gave Poppy a thorough look over. She checked her pulses, her temperature, her mucous membranes and even went to get a stethoscope from her car so she could listen to her heart. Doing something she was good at clearly helped her to feel better and the conversation became comfortable and surprisingly pleasant. She then gave Buddy a mini health check and explained different things to look out for that were specific for his breed type. It was all very useful information and it was lovely to see the real Sapna.

When she'd finished, we went to sit in the sun and had a few moments of comfortable silence.

'You know, I used to be bullied at school,' said Sapna suddenly. 'It went on for years and yet I seem to have become just like the awful girl who made my life hell. I don't know why I would do that?'

'We were talking about being bullied yesterday,' replied Jack. 'So it's a coincidence for you to say that because we actually said that you are behaving like a school bully.' She blushed and looked slightly embarrassed for having been so honest.

'I have been exactly like that,' agreed Sapna. 'I wish I knew why. Why would I want to be the person who nobody ever liked?'

'I don't know,' I answered. 'But maybe it was because you were feeling so awful from your hormones? Maybe it demonstrates how awful the bitchy girls at school must have actually been feeling? I can't imagine any balanced, happy person behaving so bloody awfully, can you?'

'That's true.' Jack nodded. 'Maybe that's what was really going on?'

'Hmmm yes, you might be right,' agreed Sapna. 'I have been feeling absolutely horrendous.'

'Why don't you take Velvet out for a little walk around the lanes?' I suggested. It's a really lovely thing to do and might help you to feel a bit happier.'

'That's a good idea,' said Sapna. 'I'm sure Velvet would enjoy that.' She stood up and called Velvet over, put her headcollar on and led her out onto the lane. It was nice to see Velvet excited as she eagerly walked out with her ears pricked up.

'Wow,' said Jack when Sapna was out of earshot. 'I can't believe that's all it took to get her to sort her mood out! Well done for opening your mouth.'

'Thanks! I think yesterday has changed me already,' I replied. 'What a relief to not have to walk on eggshells any more. I really hope the doctor can help her.'

'Me too,' agreed Jack. 'Shall we go for a ride? I think we've earned it, don't you?'

For the first time in a long time, it was deeply relaxing to leisurely groom and tack up. The ride out into the surrounding countryside was such a tonic and it was glorious to be able to enjoy the sounds of birds tweeting, cows mooing and the odd little baa. Poppy was mirroring my mood as she trotted along very happily and even laid-back Buddy had a spring in his step.

Toffee neighed as if she was saying 'Hello!' when Jack and I walked into her field to collect her, two weeks later.

'Morning ladies! Let's go into the arena.' Lynn collected another pony and led us all into the beautiful outdoor school and handed us each a pony. 'Have you been practising the mirror mantra?'

'Yes,' replied Jack. 'We've done it every day.'

'Excellent.' Lynn smiled. 'Well let's begin the session. So once again I'd like you to both walk your ponies around the arena and relax and connect with them.'

I led Toffee around the ring and chatted to her quietly about Buddy, Poppy and Velvet. Her ears pricked up at the mention of their names and she seemed to have a little smile on her face, which was nice to see.

'Ok ladies, come in to the centre and halt and then turn to face your ponies,' instructed Lynn.

We got ourselves positioned and Lynn continued.

'Now conjure up some good strong thoughts about yourselves and then send the ponies backwards by focussing behind them, lifting the lead rope and giving it a little waggle. Really look at where you want them to go and visualise light pouring out of your bellybutton pushing them backwards.'

I took a deep breath, brought my full attention to where I wanted Toffee to go and lifted the lead rope. With very little rope waggling, Toffee walked back to where I had wanted her to go. I was very pleased and surprised.

'Excellent! Well done both of you! Now focus on where your boundary line is and then invite them to walk towards you, but don't let them step over your line!'

I imagined a large, bubble of yellow light all around me. Focussed hard on exactly what I wanted Toffee to do and then invited her to walk towards me.

'And whoa,' I said firmly, putting my hand up. 'Wow! It's worked!' I was ecstatic. 'Look it worked!' I looked round to see that Jack had succeeded in halting her pony at arm's length also.

'Absolutely fantastic work! Well done!' whooped Lynn, punching the air with glee. 'You see how powerful it is when we work on ourselves? And the ponies are the best litmus test. I'm so proud of you both!'

'Tell Lynn what you did.' Jack winked.

'Ooh Grace what did you do?' asked Lynn, wide-eyed.

'Well, the day after we last saw you, I confronted Sapna! I just couldn't deal with her horrible behaviour any more.' I grinned.

'Amazing! And how did it go?' Lynn looked very impressed.

'Really good actually. She cried and apologised and then she made an appointment with her doctor to see if it was menopause making her so awful.'

'Do you know, I was going to suggest it might be the menopause making her behave so badly. It can make the nicest of people become nasty.' Lynn nodded. 'But well done for boundarying the bully. Bullies are always very weak people in reality. Only someone with deep-rooted sadness would ever behave in that way and once they are challenged, they usually wither away.' Jack and I nodded in agreement.

'So now that you have both improved your sense of self-worth and we have mastered the first step with Toffee, let's move on to step two,' Lynn continued.

The morning was full of eye-opening lessons for all of us. Toffee was a challenge as she missed her life of leisure, but I could tell that behind her resistance was a degree of interest and I was relieved that she was in the best place possible. There was no way that Jack or I could have done anything with her as she was very strong minded, and without the kind yet firm attitude from Lynn we would have all ended up very frustrated indeed.

'Lynn really knows her stuff doesn't she?' said Jack as we headed off to the carpark after the session.

'She certainly does.' I nodded. 'How lucky that Toffee can be here and get trained in such a nice way.'

'God yes. When I think of the people I've seen on YouTube "training" horses, it makes your eyes bleed. Thank the Lord you found this place, Grace.'

We got into Jack's van and drove back to our field. I looked out at all the rolling farmland and sighed with a happy heart. It was my favourite sight to see and always lifted my spirits especially on a sunny day. It finally began to sink in that I had been brave enough to challenge Sapna but in a very adult way. I hadn't just been nasty back to her, I had been calm and clear and free of the worry of her potential reaction. It was a new feeling for me and I was very pleased. My inner child was finally at peace.

If only we could be taught how to value ourselves at school, I lamented. *How many people would have a better life if they learned how to love themselves?*